D1032820

FOOT MASSAGE
AND NERVE TENSION

INA BRYANT

Illustrated

VANTAGE PRESS

NEW YORK WASHINGTON HOLLYWOOD

FIRST EDITION

Copyright © 1972, by Ina Bryant

Published by Vantage Press, Inc.
516 West 34th Street, New York, New York 10001

Manufactured in the United States of America

Standard Book No. 533-00144-7

INTRODUCTION

I am a masseuse, with a diploma from Doctor Esther Swanson's School of Swedish Massage in Chicago. All I do professionally is massage, and all it can possibly accomplish is relieve nerve tension. It is a well known fact however, that the entire body is controlled by nerves.

All my life I have read and studied authentic articles and books on the subject of the human anatomy. When my family was in the growing stage, for an hour at a session our physician conversed with me on the subject of the body and the prevention of disease. It was my privilege to study psychology in Southern Illinois Teachers College and to take a course in psychiatry from Paul von Boeckman in New York.

In grammar school and again in high school we were given a subject that was called physiology. It was an exploration of the nerves, blood vessels, glands, and other various parts of the human body. I have read a book written by Dr. Wm. H. Fitzgerald, and another by Dr. Joe Shelby Riley and W. E. Daglish, both of which were on the subject of zone therapy. It has also been my experience to sit in the classes of Eunice Ingham and hear her lecture on the use of compression massage for the feet.

In those classes she gave all due respect to the knowledge of Dr. Fitzgerald and Dr. Riley, but indicated quite a few things she had learned by doing the work. She told us she was certain there was much more yet to be discovered in the field of foot massage. Any statement about the body which may be found in this book has been acquired from the above-named sources.

CONTENTS

FOOT MASSAGE
AND NERVE TENSION

CHAPTER ONE

MASSAGE RELIEVES NERVES

Quite a few times I have been asked if there was any divine healing about this work. In the light of the previous writings of Dr. Fitzgerald and Dr. Riley, the obvious answer is that God created our bodies with this method of self-correction within them.

I would like to say that I give the complete credit to God for any or all success I have had in this field. While I labored at this massage, I constantly prayed for God to give me wisdom to use this knowledge in a way that would be beneficial to anyone with whom I have worked.

In the introduction the observation was made that Eunice Ingham in her classes indicated that she thought there was much more, probably undiscovered, in this area of work. I can truthfully say I have learned as much working professionally at foot massage as I obtained in her classes. That certainly does not discount the lectures of Eunice Ingham, because they were packed with information.

For seven years I have done foot massage in Phoenix and in the surrounding towns, administering these manipulations to more than a thousand people. Because the majority of them have asked me the same questions about this work, I am led to believe that their inquiries must be of general interest. Therefore I will give those questions and my answers to them for your consideration. Invariably the first query was: could this cure asthma, diabetes, ulcers, or whatever the particular problem happened to be.

This is a massage which relieves the nerves and allows them to function properly. Therefore anything that can be improved by normalized nerves could naturally profit thereby. In a later chapter in this book you will find quite a variety of case histories and the results reported to me after a thorough and systematic series of these massages.

I made the statement "systematic", because I firmly believe that just a little work here or there on the areas leading to problems of which people are aware is a great waste of time and the money which they are paying for the massage. More will be given on that subject in Chapter Three.

I am often asked, "If relieving my nerves does affect this problem, how many massages will it require to do the job?"

To give a definite length of time in any case is impossible because too many factors enter into the answer. The length of time they have been afflicted with this disease or discomfort can make a difference. Another circumstance in the time question is the strength of their particular physique and how rapidly they respond.

Eunice Ingham in her classes and in her writings explained that when there is an injury in the body, crystals will build at the ends of the nerves in each extremity of the nerve zone. (These nerve zones are thoroughly explained in Chapter Three.) This massage on the hands or feet reaches its ultimate goal when it has, by means of manipulations, cracked the crystals enough so that the blood can dissolve them and then the person no longer has them.

So long as those crystals are hanging there, they act on the nerves like a short in a light circuit. When the blood has disposed of them, the nerves are released to function properly. Out of more than a thousand people, one man's feet were cleared of the crystals in one massage. Another man's feet responded on the third, and still another on the fourth.

So many feet were freed from crystals at six, eight, ten, twelve, fourteen, and on up to eighteen and twenty massages. The only way I could give the exact number would be to go back through my books and count them case by case. I do remember that one woman cleared at thirty-eight, and another at sixty-eight. They stand out in my mind because I worked with them for so long.

I also recall a man whose feet I massaged twice a week for fifteen months. I would have quit; but he would not relinquish the hope that some day he would feel nothing but my thumb and fingers going over his feet. At last, after a year and three months, the day came.

Often he said to me, "I do not regret one penny I've paid you. The results in my body have been well worth it. I could not hear anything out of my left ear, and now there is no more noise in it and I can hear as well with it as with the other ear. My back gave me constant agony, and now it feels wonderful. There are lots of ways I am better."

The mention of crystals always evokes the following questions. "What does a crystal look like? How do I know they are there? Do you feel them?"

They mean, do I, the masseuse, feel them as I massage the foot. No, I do not feel them. A few times I have felt something crackling under my thumb which resembled the breaking of thin ice, but I would not say it was the crystals.

I have never seen one of the crystalline deposits; but a woman whom I know told me that an osteopath operated on her finger to remove a gout crystal. He gave a local anesthetic, cut in and picked it out with a pair of tweezers. She watched him. And she told me it had the appearance of isinglass.

In answer to the question, "How can I know the crystals are there?"

You will know that something is there by the way it feels. Sometimes the massage on the feet will cause a feeling as if needles were prickling, or a fingernail file jabbing, or a fingernail half an inch long cutting, or a darning needle digging. One man said it felt more like a pitchfork prong plunging in.

At this point I can just hear someone say, "Ugh, I could never take that."

A good masseur or masseuse watches your face to see how much pain you are feeling and to hold it to an endurable point. I often tell people that this is a peculiar massage, for which they pay me to hurt them, so I must make them feel pain.

It is a strange fact, but children will beg for these manipulations when they know they are going to hurt. When I have finished the first foot massage on people, they will invariably remark something to the effect it makes their feet feel so good. They also marvel that anything which hurts like that can be so relaxing to the nerves all over the body.

What you feel is caused by the manner in which the crystal has been broken when it strikes against the nerve. There is one sensation that I have not yet mentioned. I believe it can best be described by Figure I.

I was massaging a man's foot when he flinched and said it felt as if I had touched a live wire to his toe. I was working along the area indicated in Figure I by Line I. He felt the electrical shock at Point 2 in Figure I.

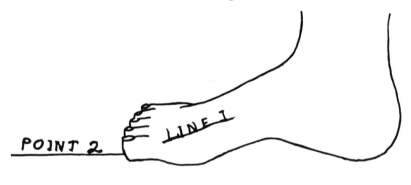

Fig. 1

Many times those whose feet I was massaging have told me they felt something that resembled a light electrical shock. After feeling the sensations which have been described, and then the massage gives you nothing more than an awareness the thumb or finger of the masseuse is passing over your foot, you can rest assured there are no crystals left.

14

One man, when he first felt the sharpness in his foot as I massaged, said, "This is amazing." The tenth routine, his feet were yet full of various pains. The eleventh, he felt nothing but the light pressure of my thumb and fingers. Again he said, "This is most amazing."

"I told you," I reminded him.

"I know you told me, but I didn't believe you," and he laughed. His mother and I had been very good friends throughout her lifetime. He had known and trusted me many years before I started this work.

Dr. Fitzgerald and Dr. Riley advocated the use of clothespins clamped on the fingers and toes; but Eunice Ingham told her class that too much pressure for a long time was injurious to the little nerves. Because of things people have reported to me, I am firmly convinced that crystals can be built at the end of the nerves by too much massage.

I had taught a woman to do these manipulations on her own feet. One day she called me and said that her back was simply killing her. When I asked if she was massaging her feet, she told me she was doing it faithfully every day. I had told her twice a week, but she had not heeded.

This time I emphasized, "Stop it every day. You must be building crystals."

In two weeks she called me to say that she had dropped back to twice a week and that her back had entirely quit hurting.

Another frequent question is, "Will my problem be gone when the crystals have disappeared?" For the answer to that I would like to give you the case histories of a few people.

C. R. came to me with a situation from which he had suffered for twenty years. It was growing rapidly worse. He told me his seventh cervical had slipped to the right. Three good chiropractors had told him that the bone would break before it would go back into position because it was set in calcium.

He was suffering from headaches, dizziness, and what he

described as "feeling like a hard wind blowing out at one ear." He could not lift his hands as high as his shoulders, and he could not turn his head to either side.

I gave him five foot massages. When he came back for the sixth, he told me he had no headache, no dizziness, and no hard wind blowing out at one ear. He said he could turn his head normally, and put his hands behind his shoulders. When I went over his feet that time, he felt nothing but the light pressure of my fingers.

He asked me, "How in the world could you rub my feet and make a bone move which the chiropractors could not even push? It had to move because I could feel it sticking out over there on the right side, and now it is even with the other vertebra."

I explained that on his thyroid gland were four little parathyroid glands. Their chief duty in the body is to distribute calcium where it belongs. When they are restrained from their proper function by inactive nerves, calcium can be deposited where it does not belong.

When the crystals in his feet had been cracked enough so that the blood could dissolve them, the hindrance to that section of his nerves had thus been removed. In turn the nerves had directed the parathyroid glands, and they had simply performed their normal duty by removing the calcium from the seventh cervical to its proper location in the body.

Furthermore, the purpose of the muscles and tendons surrounding the vertebra is to hold them in their correct position. If the vertebra is slipped a little (I am speaking of situations which a good chiropractor has told me can happen) the normal thing would be for the muscles and tendons to draw the bone back into its correct arrangement.

It has been previously stated that the nerves are shorted by the crystals so they cannot function at their best. Consequently in this case they would not direct and the muscles would not pull. When the crystalline deposits were gone and the nerves liberated, they then began their proper con-

16

trol of the muscles. The muscles thus prompted pulled the bone into line.

C. R. told me that while the bone was going back the feeling of a wind blowing out at one ear was so terrible that he thought he could not bear it. He made himself go to bed —and went right to sleep. The next morning all that discomfort was gone.

As I have stated in the introduction, all I do is massage and it gives relief from nerve tension. The body does the rest. One man had what the doctors called a whiplash neck injury. He had pain in his neck, back, one arm, and in one leg. He said he had been given one hundred and forty adjustments by chiropractors and osteopaths, but all to no avail.

For six months he had done nothing in the way of treatments. He had decided he must suffer for the rest of his life. Three of these massages, and he said his pain was all gone, and he felt no crystals in his feet.

The case history of R. O. will show the difference in the same body between a fresh and an old injury. He said he had wrenched his back at work the day before. When he came to me he walked as if he might be a hundred. He could hardly get up, and he could not get down without groaning. Every movement, as he expressed it, was agony.

I gave him the complete routine on his feet, and he went home. Three hours later he told his wife his back hurt worse than before I had massaged his feet. She reminded him that I had said he might have a reaction. He thought if he was having a reaction it must be a healthy one.

The next time I saw R. O. He told me his back hurt him much worse after the massage until about noon the next day, when it began to feel better. Within forty-eight hours he declared every particle of the pain was gone.

He was really excited. "Let's see what you can do with this old chronic condition between my shoulders. My hands are always going numb, and the chiropractor says it is from vertebra in my back."

I gave him fourteen thorough routines on his feet, but he said there was no use to go any further because it was not going to do anything for this. If I had known then what I know now I would have tried to get him to continue, but at that time I did not blame him for being discouraged. The work with him was discontinued.

Six months later he came and said that since he had received those fourteen routines on his feet, his back and hands had been better than at any time since they had begun to bother him. He had not had any other kind of treatment and he was certain that the massage had made the change.

Three months after that he came and asked me to give him some more foot massages. Eight more routines of the manipulations were administered, and his feet seemed to be cleared of the crystals. Two years afterward he told me that the problem with his back and hands had completely disappeared, and he was certain the foot massages were responsible. He said he had suffered far too many years before he came to me to believe it would have gone away without assistance.

R. O. was a much younger man than C. R. and yet his chronic condition required twenty-two massages. C. R. had suffered from the calcified seventh cervical for twenty years, but six of the very same manipulations given to R. O., and C. R. was liberated from both crystals and distress.

Another man affected with bursitus in a shoulder and having a heart ailment felt nothing but the pressure on his feet the fourth massage. He said he had stopped his pain pills and forgotten his bursitus, and his heart had ceased to bother him. His wife, who had assured me there was very little wrong with her, required sixteen of the same massages to set her feet free from the crystals.

These histories should explain the reason I could never predict for anyone how many times I must massage their feet before the crystals will be gone. These cases should also answer the question as to whether the problem will be solved when the feet feel nothing but my fingers. In four of these people the pain was not present when the crystals were gone, but with one the pain did not leave until about six months later.

After four or five years of this work, I counted to see what type of report had been given in each case. Ninety percent had told me they were well pleased with the results they felt in their bodies. Some of the other ten percent said their problem had dissolved six months later.

CHAPTER TWO

NUTRITION, EMOTIONS, AND UNUSUAL
SITUATIONS AS CONNECTED WITH FOOT MASSAGE

Since foot massage is a means by which the body can re-adjust itself it would naturally follow that nutrition is a most important factor in the length of time required for the crystals to leave the feet even though they may have been sufficiently cracked. That our foods are lacking in proper nourishment is a fact which has been discussed by even our government officials.

When I tell people how important correct nourishment is to the success of the work, they invariably begin to ask me what they should eat. I always stress that I am a masseuse and not a dietician or an authority on nutrition. There are reputable nutrition centers, with qualified managers. On request, they will be glad to recommend some valuable writings on the subject.

However, I have found a few things which seem to help tremendously with those whose crystals stay in the feet in spite of many massages. Once I had worked with three members of a family when I was asked to begin the routine on the feet of the fourth, who was the mother.

I had given her the manipulations twice a week for a month when she told me that just before I had begun with her, her gynecologist had informed her that she must not wait longer than three months to have a complete hysterectomy. He said that her female organs were at the stage just before malignancy.

I asked her why she did not try the advice of Jethro Kloss.

In his book, *Back To Eden*, he made the statement that red-clover-blossom tea was a must in a case of cancer. He stressed the importance of drinking it instead of water. In that book he also said he had cured one internal cancer with golden-seal tea alone.

The golden-seal tea was bitter, and she refused it; but she did drink the red-clover-blossom beverage. Using one big handful of the dried blossoms to half a gallon of water from the tap, she put it on the stove and allowed it to reach almost the boiling point but not quite. Keeping the container tightly covered, it was removed from the fire and allowed to steep until it was entirely cooled. That required two or three hours.

She then strained it into a gallon jar and finished filling the vessel with water thus diluting the tea to twice the amount. That was placed in the refrigerator. From it she took a good drink as often as she remembered which, she told me, amounted to perhaps six or eight large glasses a day.

When I gave her the twelfth massage on her feet she felt no crystals cracking. She told me that the week before she had gone to her gynecologist for an examination before he would put her in the hospital for the hysterectomy. The day before I had come this last time, he had called her to report on the last tests he had made.

He had said, "I have good news for you. You not only do not have any malignancy, but you have no problem at all now."

You can imagine the joy of her family, to say nothing of herself. Furthermore, the experience had given me an idea. To have had as much sharpness as was apparent in her feet when I began with her, the crystals had disappeared in a comparatively short time.

After that, when someone went on with massage after massage for a long period of time, I would suggest they try drinking the red-clover-blossom tea. There were exceptions, but usually they began to improve almost immediately.

I have no idea what is in the blossoms, but this I do know: I was raised on a farm in southern Illinois. We would never think of beginning the winter months without our barn loft full of red-clover hay, which included the dried blossoms. This was prepared for food for our cattle, and we never had such a thing as a sick cow. All winter those cows rewarded us with gallons and gallons of rich milk. Never once did the idea enter our minds that the clover was good food for us also.

Often when I suggested to a person whose feet I was massaging that it might be well if they would consult someone on the subject of nutrition, they asked me what I ate. Many people express amazement that at seventy years of age I can still work as many hours as I do.

They often ask, "Where do you get your strength?"

Because so many people have inquired concerning my diet, it might be well to give it here. I am definitely not prescribing it, or urging it, or even recommending it. I am simply stating that this is what I eat.

My son came from another state to visit me. Because I had company, I had collected a supply of foods I do not eat. When he came to breakfast the first morning, I asked him what he wanted to eat and began to name some of the things I had bought especially because he was there.

He asked, "What are you going to eat?"

I told him he did not want what I ate.

He said, "Prepare me the same as you are going to eat, and see what I do."

I prepared it, and he ate. He went back home and told his wife, "Anything that can give a woman of Mother's age the energy she has, I'm all for it."

I can also say that I used to be the easiest person in the world to be sick with everything contagious that came my way. Now, in my work, I am among all kinds of diseases, such as the latest in virus, and I never have an attack unless I do not get my proper hours of sleep. If you are wondering what I call correct time for slumber, again I am not speaking of anyone else. I am simply saying I function best at my present age with nine hours out of each twenty-four.

My Menu

Breakfast

1 teaspoon of chia seeds	seeds
1 teaspoon of alfalfa seeds	2 tablespoons of steamed
3 tablespoons of sunflower	brown rice
seeds	1½ tablespoons of sesame
2 tablespoons of pumpkin	seed butter

I thoroughly mix the above items, and then I chew and chew and chew.

Dinner

Which is eaten at noon instead of at night. Two cooked vegetables with a cup of sprouted lentils sprinkled over them. Sometimes I eat a wheat cake, which is not really a pastry but is made from sprouted wheat.

Last Meal Of The Day

Fruit—raw or cooked, or often just the unsweetened organic juice such as cherry, apple, or grape. In addition to the above I use one food supplement, but no vitamins.

Often I am asked how to sprout the lentils and wheat.

Measure a third or fourth of the desired amount of the sprouted grain or legume, because both will swell. Cover with water to at least three or four inches above that which is being sprouted, and allow to stand all night.

The next morning pour off the water but leave in a deep bowl or, better than that, a plastic colander. Wash three or four times a day by holding it under the faucet and allowing the water to run through. After it is washed it can be set in a pie pan or dish on the workshelf. When the sprouts are half an inch long, wash well and place in the refrigerator.

The sprouted grain or legume loses its starch and becomes rich in vitamins, according to writers on the subject. The wheat cake I mentioned has the appearance of a soggy cake but is not a pastry.

Sprouted Wheat Cake

2 cups sprouted wheat	4 tablespoons of sesame seed
4 tablespoons of raw sugar or	oil
honey	1 teaspoon salt
	1 doz. eggs

Blend in osterizer. Pour into a well-oiled shallow baking dish. Bake at 275° temperature.

I drink no coffee, cokes, or tea except red-clover-blossom tea which I use instead of water. I try to follow some advice I once read. Eat like a king for breakfast, like a poor man at noon, and a pauper at night.

Emotions And The Foot Massages

I believe it is safe to make the assertion that emotions prevent the feet from losing the crystals after the massages more than any other one thing. I am also convinced that anger should head the list.

I had given these massages for quite awhile to one man. His feet would seem to be better, then worse, then better again. I began to probe for a solution.

When I mentioned anger, he laughed. "I don't get angry," he said. "I just plainly have mad fits."

I explained that passion injured the body and built crystals while he was paying me to massage them out. He agreed to stop, and we were really making progress. It appeared that one more routine on his feet, and he would feel nothing but my thumb and fingers. To my surprise, the next time his feet were as bad as when the first massage was given.

"Now what's the matter?" He was really disgusted.

I asked, "Charley, have you—"

"Yes, I have. Twice today. These dumb people—"

He expanded on the stupidity of the average human with whom he came in contact in his business.

"Charley, these people are not going to consider your problems or even worry about them. Either you have to cope with the public and keep yourself calm, or I never can get your feet free from crystals."

He decided, then, we might as well stop at once. In order to live, he had to keep his business. According to him, he could not manage it properly and hold his temper. The last I heard from him he had just undergone an operation. I had learned to have a strong feeling for him and his wife, but he had limited my ability to help him.

Once I was giving a woman a massage, and she felt sharpness in only two or three places. We decided that one more would end her need of me, but the next time her feet were full of crystals. When I asked what had taken place to upset her peace of mind, her story came tumbling out.

Her first grandchild was three or four weeks old, and her son's wife did not know the first thing about caring for a baby. She would grab up the poor little dear and allow its head to wobble about with no support. She realized that a mother-in-law must keep her mouth shut, but that baby was her own flesh and blood. What in the world was she going to do?

I told her about another mother-in-law whose daughter-in-law did not know a thing in the world about caring for her child. That mother-in-law had wept.

Her youngest son, who was still at home, had said, "Don't cry, Mother. If God wants that baby to live it will survive in spite of her."

That baby became a grown woman.

This grandmother had a sense of humor and was laughing. She decided she could worry herself into her grave and not do the grandchild a particle of good. She would have to turn her head and not look, and pray for the mercy of God to save it.

The next massage she felt no sharpness in her feet. Many other examples could be given, but this should stress the fact that emotions must be controlled to the best of our ability.

WARNING

I have read about and have heard people say that we can massage feet with confidence because no one could be hurt by these manipulations. I knew a woman who died in a car accident and yet she was not injured. The doctors decided it came about because the shock was too great for her nerves and her heart, which had previously given no problem, succumbed under the strain.

I am convinced that some precautions should be considered. Do not give these massages for at least three weeks after an operation. I do not administer them to a pregnant woman, unless she has been having them before she became pregnant. I do not give a foot massage to anyone directly under a doctor's care without consulting him whether it meets with his approval.

Do not give these manipulations to an asthmatic, a diabetic, or a person who is subject to angina attacks, until after you have thoroughly considered the reports of some people who were suffering from these ailments and were given the foot massages. These cases are discussed in Chapters 9, 10, and 11.

When every area of a foot is quite painful as the crystals crack, it is best to be certain that the massage does not become more than those particular nerves can accept. If the person suddenly feels chilly, stop the work immediately. It sometimes requires several attempts before some individuals can tolerate a complete massage over the entire areas of both feet.

There was the case of a young girl. When her parents came to talk to me they wept as they told me about their sixteen-year-old daughter. All her life she had been sick and no one had been able to give them a reasonable solution as to why she was so nervous and morose. Her mother had caught her in the nick of time once as she was preparing to take an overdose of sleeping pills in an attempt to end it all.

At last the doctors had despaired and told them to take her to a psychiatrist. The parents said that the more he talked to her, the worse she became. He said she was not trying to help herself, and his advice was to have her take shock treatments at a state hospital. The mere thought of her being there when she was so young broke their hearts. Anxiously they asked if the foot massages could help.

Naturally they had to be given the only answer there was. Massage was acknowledged as giving relief to tense nerves. No promises could be made. If they wanted her to try it, I would do my best. They admitted they were grabbing at straws. They would try it.

The manipulations were begun on the big toe of her right foot. The toes were not half completed when her behavior became such that everything on the foot was stopped. It appeared that she was going to lose all self-control.

She was asked to lie on her bed and a little effleurage and petrisage were given around her head and neck. These were done with a very light touch. In a few minutes she was sleeping soundly under my hands, and I tiptoed out of the room. Her mother said she had a long restful nap, and when she awakened she was quite calm. She told her mother that what had just been done to her was better than any sleeping pill she had ever taken, and she wanted more.

We continued with a little more work on her feet each time until she could tolerate no more. Then the Swedish was given on her head and neck to put her to sleep. It was six weeks of this, twice a week, before she could accept the complete routine on her feet.

At last came the day when she did not require the Swedish on her head and neck. It was then that her mother told me that she had quit all nerve and sleeping pills. She also said it was the sweetest sound she had ever heard the first time that girl giggled with the freedom of others of her age. The last I heard from her, she was in high school and doing quite well.

Unusual Situations

Because of diabetes, one woman had suffered the amputation of half of each foot. In the stump of one foot she had an ulcer that was all of two inches across, and so deep that a bone could be detected at the bottom. The only place she could be given the massage was on her hands. The cracking of the crystals in them created so much pain it was quite some time before she could accept the complete routine.

This woman told me she had not been without a daily shot of insulin for twenty-three years; but after the compression massage was begun, she was forced to stop because she would have gone into insulin shock. She said she was positive that her pancreas had begun to secrete its own insulin. She also showed me that the big ulcer had completely healed. She said she was convinced that the hand massages were responsible for all of it.

In a person with both hands and feet the massage should be done on the feet, but there are a few exceptions. If the feet are incapacitated for any reason, it is best to try the hands.

When I was quite new in this work, a polio victim called for me. She had suffered an attack when she was five years of age and had never been able to take another step. She was now in her fifties, and all day long she pulled herself about in a wheelchair because she was a busy woman. Her hands and arms were well developed and strong. but her feet hung in helpless inactivity. Being new in the foot massage, and believing that if the feet were there it must be done on them, that was my first approach to the work on her.

She felt very little of the cracking of the crystals, and no results in her body. I decided to try the hands. She said there was a high degree of sharpness in those big strong hands, and later reported two very definite changes in her body.

Ever since the polio her back had pained her day and night, week in and week out. She had been everywhere she could find any therapy for polio-suffering people, including the Sister Kenny, but all to no avail. After something like a dozen of massages on her hands she said she was completely relieved of the continuous grinding pain in her back.

She also said that something came from her in the urine. She described it as resembling small ice crystals which were amber-colored. Simultaneously with this, her sides became quite sore in the area where she had been previously told the ureter tubes passed from the kidneys to the bladder. Later she reported there were no more amber-colored crystals and that all soreness had gone from her sides.

Another time, it appears, the work should be done on the hands instead of the feet is when too much discomfort develops in the feet after the massages. I am not speaking of minor distress with the lower extremeties, such as little sharp shooting pains which subside after twenty-four hours or of soreness if it soon disappears.

One man said that every time he was given the routine on his feet, for a day or two they would feel so sore it was uncomfortable to push on the pedals of his car. He was always certain that I had bruised them, but he could never find the slightest discoloration and within twenty-four to forty-eight hours all the soreness would be gone and his feet felt wonderful.

As already asserted, we are not referring to cases like that but rather to something much more drastic. A woman from California had been in Arizona long enough for me to do eighteen massages on her feet. She assured me that her blood pressure was down to normal, and her nerves were much improved, but her feet were quite a problem. She said they were sore and swollen. But at that time she went back home, so there was nothing I could do.

Three months later she returned. All that time she had suffered with sore, badly swollen and inflamed feet. She had been to a doctor, who had sent her to a foot specialist. Nothing had relieved her. She could not wear an ordinary shoe, and could barely endure the pressure of the lightest and softest house slippers that could be found. She had come back to Arizona to get me to massage her feet.

After looking at her feet I refused to touch them, but insisted on doing the work on her hands. She contended that it would not do her any good. The only reason she finally agreed was because she saw that I was not going to massage her feet when they were in that condition.

After the first manipulations on her hands, she declared that her feet felt better. After six thorough routines on the hands, she said that all swelling, inflammation and soreness were gone from her feet and she was going back home to California.

She told everyone with whom she discussed this massage that no one would ever give manipulations on her feet again. It had to be done on her hands. She said if her feet started swelling, she would be back. That was four or five months ago, and I have not heard from her.

Mrs. D. is an entirely different story. She had been given some foot massages some few months previously and declared there was nothing like it so far as she was concerned. Although she was eighty, she vowed she felt much younger after the work on her feet.

One day she called and said she was just barely able to walk. She wanted me to come and give her some more foot massages. I found that she had developed some very tender red spots on her feet which her doctor had told her might become ulcers.

He had given her medicine to put on the spots, and told her to stay off of her feet. She felt that to quit walking at her age might end activity for her. Also the sitting and the medicine did not improve the problem in the least. She thought that if anything, they were becoming worse.

The spots were so numerous that nothing could be done on the feet without touching them. As the other woman had done, Mrs. D. argued. She was certain she could get no results from the hands. Knowing my position as a masseuse, and the danger of massaging over areas that were inflamed, I utterly refused to work on her feet.

After six routines on the hands, Mrs. D. told me that every red spot had vanished and she was really on her feet again. She, like the other woman, said that from this experience she was convinced that from there on it was nothing but the hands for her.

Mrs. H. and her husband gave me some reports that were really astounding even to me, who had already been told much exciting news about experiences within bodies after these manipulations on the feet and hands.

One Friday morning Mrs. H. fell from a chair on which she was standing. Her heelbone was broken in three pieces, and one section was driven up and wedged into the bones above it so tightly that the doctor told Mr. H. they could not draw it down with a clamp. They would have to cut in and pull it down. They would not do that immediately because they feared that the broken bone might have cut into the blood line.

If the blood line had been severed, there would be no

point in even setting the bone because it could never heal; the only answer would be to amputate the foot. She had also broken a toe, and a bone in the middle of the same foot. The doctor told Mr. H. that if she ever did walk on that foot again it would be at least three months.

As soon as Mr. H. had his wife in the hospital, she asked him to find me. As I was out at work, he was not able to contact me until five o'clock that evening. He knew I could do nothing in the hospital, but he said she just wanted to talk to me.

Mrs. H. wanted me to tell her which spot on the hand corresponded to the heelbone. She realized they would not allow me to do the foot massage in the hospital, but there was nothing to prevent her from massaging her own hand as best she could. When I simply touched the place on her hand, it was quite tender.

You will find that space designated in Figure 8, Chapter Three, under the foot. It was her right heelbone which was broken. On Wednesday the heel was again X-rayed and they found nothing to do but put the foot in a cast. Mrs. H. said they gave her no anesthetic, and she lay there and watched.

When she came home from the hospital, they called for me. The massage was done on the right hand and left foot. In six weeks from the time of the accident, Mr. and Mrs. H. went on a trip and she walked with not even so much as a cane. It was quite a relief to them, for the verdict had been that if she ever walked again it would be at least three months.

The question has been asked, "Will exercise crack these crystals?"

My husband, who has a mechanical mind, has always thought that some machine should be invented to do the job. Exercise is always good, but nothing will crack these crystals without damage to the tiny nerves to which they are attached like the human thumb or finger. Also the mani-

32

pulation that will break them in one part of the same foot will not work the correct way in another area.

When I first began this work, I despaired about some people because I could not make them feel the cracking of the crystals. Later, I decided I was wrong to quit trying. I had been told that if there was a problem in the body, there were crystals in the feet. If that was true, then it was up to me, the masseuse, to find some way to break them. That was when I evolved two manipulations of which I had never heard. They are described and given in Figure 24 and Figure 25, Chapter Four.

Often the question is asked, "Why do the crystals build when there is an injury to the body?"

I have no answer except that God made it that way.

CHAPTER THREE

EXPLANATION OF ZONES

For those who may have never read an explanation of zones, I will give a brief summary. Remember, we are speaking of zones and not of nerves or nervous systems. A zone begins at the thumb of the right hand and goes up the arm, up the neck, and to the top of the head, then back down the backbone, the leg, and on to the big toe of the right foot.

Another zone starts with the forefinger of the right hand and proceeds beside the first one in the same manner to the top of the head, back down the body and the same leg to the toe next to the big one on the right foot. The third zone starts with the second finger, and follows the same course beside the second zone down to the second little toe.

I have been massaging a toe when the party receiving the manipulations would tell me that the corresponding finger "tingled." One time, after a complete foot massage, the woman on whom the work was done held her hands up and called attention to the fact that they were fiery red. No part of her anatomy had been touched but the feet.

Figure 2 shows a diagram which I have drawn to illustrate the zones as I understood them after hearing them explained in a class. In the introduction to this book, I told where I derived all my information about the body. To the best of my knowledge, Figure 2 does not duplicate any previous diagram or drawing. Since there is only one system of nerve zones in the body, it might be similar.

When I began this work I used the charts of the woman from whom I learned. Gradually I began to wonder if there

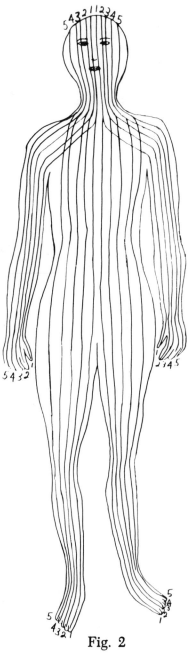

Fig. 2

were not areas which no one had discovered. I was giving the massages to two women who did not know each other, but both had severe problems with their eyes. Neither reported any improvement. At that time I was, as previously stated, massaging for the eyes on areas designated on charts already published by others. The eye areas on them are given in Figure 3.

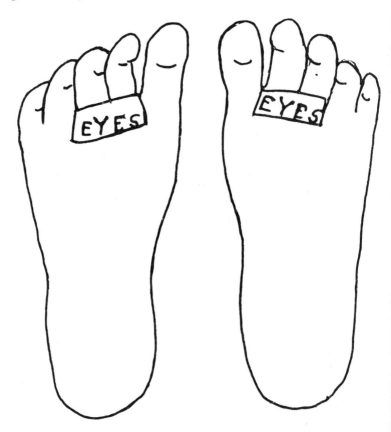

After massaging thoroughly, and neither woman had reported improvement, I decided to try around the roots of the same toes where they joined the top of the foot. Inside of two weeks, both women were telling me that their eyes were definitely better.

From that time on I began to try other and more lines and spots for various problems people told me they had. I could mention case after case of people who told me things which caused me to add to my routine. I will simply make the statement that Figures 4, 5, 6, 7, 8, 9 and 10 will designate all the areas I covered in the foot massages, because people told me they received decided improvement after that particular part of the foot or hand had received the manipulations.

I can truthfully say that more than a thousand people, whose feet and hands I have rubbed, have helped me to make the following charts from the accounts of the responses of their bodies. I have simply compiled their reports and drawn the figures to illustrate them.

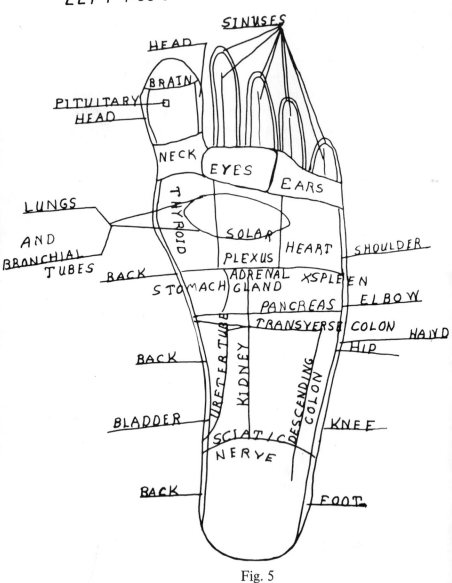

Fig. 5

38

RIGHT FOOT

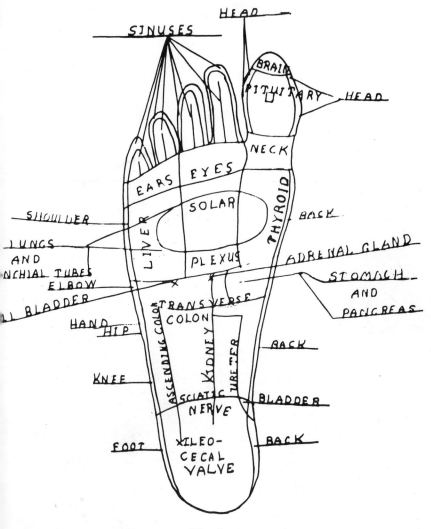

Fig. 4

39

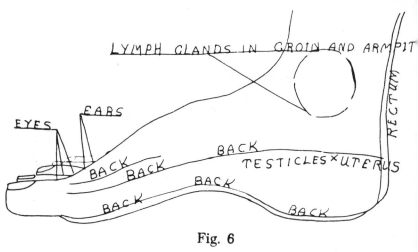

Fig. 6

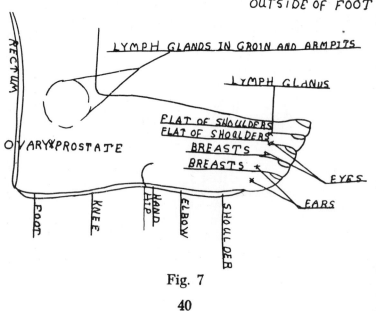

Fig. 7

40

PALM OF RIGHT HAND

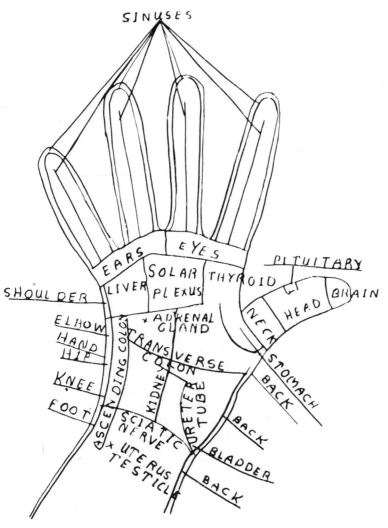

Fig. 8

PALM OF LEFT HAND

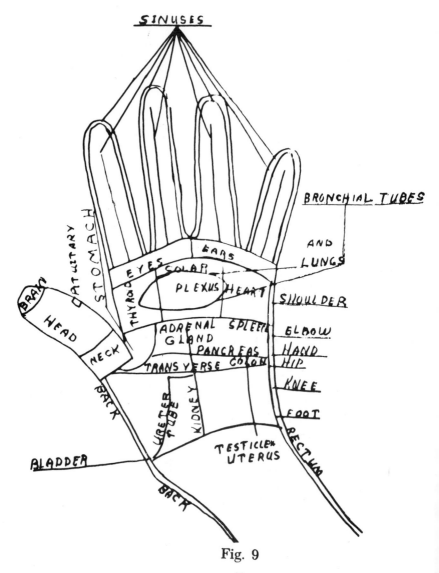

Fig. 9

42

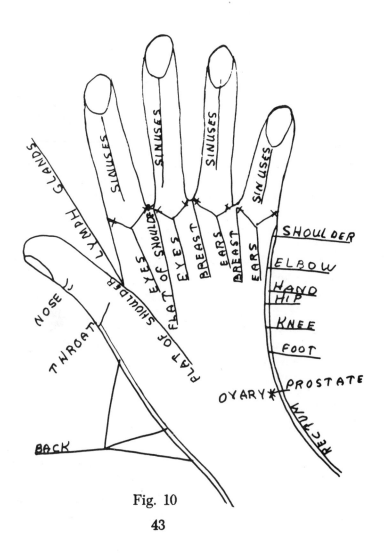

BACK OF RIGHT AND LEFT HANDS ARE
ARE THE SAME

Fig. 10

43

Chapter Four

THE ACTUAL WORK

Although this chapter will be dealing with the actual massage, I urge you not to begin until you have read and thoroughly studied Chapters Nine, Ten, and Eleven. Since Dr. Fitzgerald and Dr. Riley firmly believed that each part of the body was represented in the feet, no area should be neglected.

Once I met a woman whose daughter told me that her mother thought she had heart trouble. She had gone through every test and examination including a cardiograph, but nothing like that could be found. However, the woman dropped dead within a few weeks. The decision from the postmortem examination was that she had died from a heart attack.

All of us have heard of similar cases, where the person had undergone a thorough physical examination and was pronounced free from some particular problem in the body. Later, that same person was found to have the specific ailment which had not been previously located. That shows us beyond a doubt that our bodies can be building something which we do not yet feel, or even suspect from the best and most accurate tests.

It has been stressed in previous writings of others that the crystals are built at the ends of the zones when the body suffers an injury; if there is no trouble in the body, there are no crystals in the feet. If this is true, then why not know what is in that foot on which you are doing the manipulations? It appears sensible, logical, and humanitarian not to neglect a single area whether it is on the feet of a customer who is paying you to free his nerves, or if it is a member of your family.

To avoid missing any part of the foot where the crystals might be lurking, I made myself a routine to follow. When a foot feels nothing but my thumb and fingers going over it, the satisfaction is mine that the nerves of the recipient have really been set free. The good reports afterward have verified the belief in a thorough system of massage.

As previously stated in this book, it sometimes becomes necessary to work on the hands. Therefore I have also evolved a method of procedure on them, which will be given in Chapter Five.

I begin with the right foot, and do not go over any line less than three times or more than four. As shown in Figure II, begin with three lines up the outside of the big toe from where it joins the foot to the end of the toe.

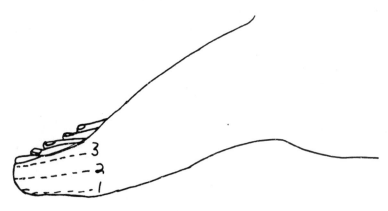

Fig. 11

It is most important that the thumb or finger being used in the manipulation snuggles closely against the toe. That is to make certain that every curve in or out on the toe receives the same even massage. If you begin at the bottom of the line where the toe joins the foot in the average case, it is necessary to stand the thumb or finger on end in order to be thorough with the first deep curve.

Next, do three lines up the inside of the same big toe from the base, where it joins the foot up to the end. The first one of these lines will be close to the bottom side of the big toe. The second line is in the middle of the inside of the toe. The third is still on the inside but next to the top of the toe.

As shown in Figure 12 by dots No. 1, work across the big toe where it joins the foot. As indicated in Figure 12 by dots No. 2, manipulate along a line at the joint underneath the big toe. As given in Figure 12 by dots No. 3, massage across the end of the big toe.

On top of the same big toe do Lines 1 and 2 as marked in Figure 13.

Next is the pituitary area, which is in the middle of the flat of the same big toe as shown on Figure 4. It is difficult to massage correctly because the toe flattens out, and the nerve with the crystals at the end of it slides over the inside of the toe. The manipulation begins with the thumb against the inside as shown in Picture A.

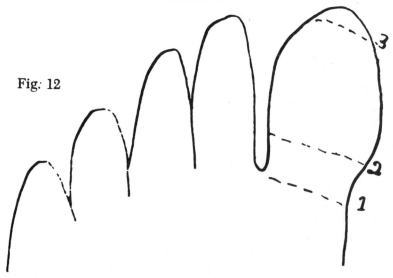

Fig: 12

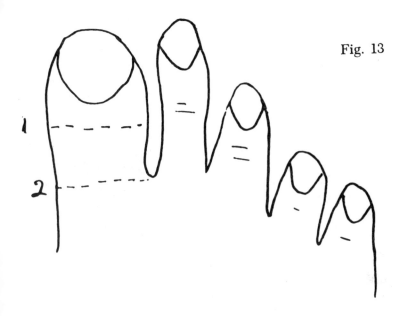

Fig. 13

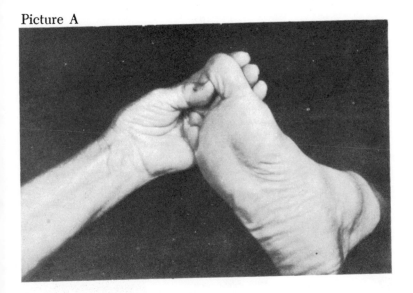

Picture A

47

Slowly, until you learn this, move the thumb toward the middle of the flat of the big toe with firm (not hard) even pressure in such a way as to carry the end of the nerve with the crystals attached into the center of the flat of the toe as shown in Picture B.

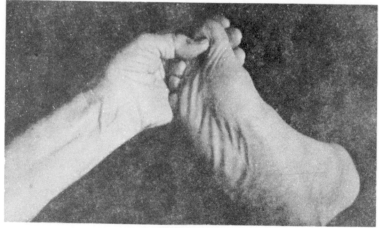

Picture B

When the position in Picture B is reached, give a little quick motion using the joint in the middle of the thumb in such a way as to stand the thumb on a corner of the end and crack the crystals as shown in Picture C.

Picture C

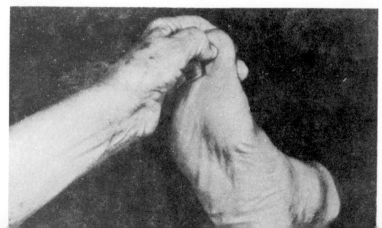

If the person on whose toe you are working, as shown in Pictures A, B, and C feels discomfort when your thumb is standing on end, you have done the manipulation well. You can rest assured that you have cracked the crystals in that area. Repeat the flexing of the thumb three times.

If the person feels nothing but the pressure of your thumb, either there is no crystal or you have failed to carry it and the nerve back into the correct position for the thumb to crack it.

In the latter case, go back to the beginning of the description of working the pituitary area, and carefully follow the instructions given in the Pictures A. B, and C.

As shown by the dots in Figure 14, begin at the very root of the first smaller toe on its side, next to the big toe, and

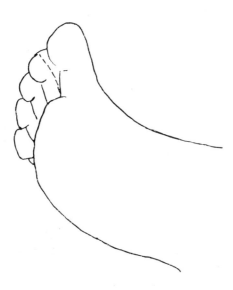

Fig. 14

work a line up and into the tip of the toe.

All toes are not exactly the same. In some, you will find the line a little toward the front of the middle line in the side. In others, it may be slightly toward the back; but more often it will be exactly as designated by the dots in Figure 14.

Massage in a similar way on the opposite side of the same toe from the bottom up, and meet the line, as shown in Figure 14, at the very top end of the toe.

Next, underneath the same toe, work from where it joins the foot, up and into the center of the pad of the toe, as shown by dots in Figure 15.

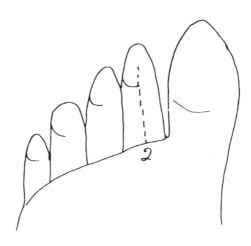

Fig. 15

The dots in Figure 15 denote a line that is not usually easy to follow, especially if the toe is skinny and the pad thick. You will often find this. You must work very carefully up the bony toe, and right under the thick pad. Slowly and carefully come on up the plump surface and into the center where the line ends.

If this is not well done, crystals will be left untouched to grow where the line springs out from the skinny toe onto the thick pad. If you will notice this in Figure 4, you will realize how important these particular lines of massage are to those suffering from sinus conditions.

As the dots in Figure 16 indicate, work a line on top of the same toe from the base of the toe, up to the nail, or vice versa. On the other three smaller toes use the same routine for the first one. Because of the necessity of such a detailed description of this work on the toes, you might be discouraged and think it would take ages to simply do the toes. But that is not true.

It is not half so difficult as the lengthy instruction would seem to indicate. In fact after you have become thoroughly

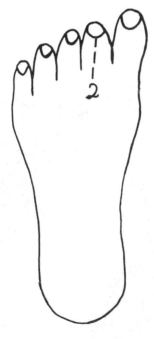

Fig. 16

acquainted with these manipulations and this part of the routine, you can easily finish all the toes, including the big one, in less than five minutes.

The next part of the routine is to begin at the base of the little toe, underneath, and. work around each toe where it joins the foot and in between, moving along toward but not including the big toe. If you remember, this was included in the massage on the big toe. In some cases the crystals crack better by coming from the big toe back to the little one.

The only way to know is to try to find out what the recipient feels most in his foot. As you may have read in Chapter One, when the crystals crack they may feel like a needle prickling, a fingernail jabbing, a thorn, an electrical shock, or just plain soreness. It might be simply a pain, sharp or dull. Sometimes the crystals crack more easily if the thumb of the left hand is used to work along this line in the way shown in Picture D.

With another foot it may require the use of the right thumb, moving from next to the big toe, around the base of

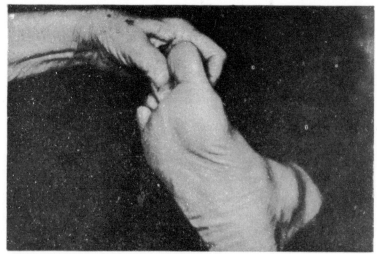

Picture D

each toe, and in between as you move toward the little toe. This is done with the hand up and the thumb on end. If there is no definite feeling that the crystals are cracking as you massage in this fashion, then with the left hand below, and the left thumb reaching up, and the joint bent in such a way as to bring the corner of the thumb down around the base of the little toe, continue toward the big toe. Do not despair until you have tried every possible manupilation.

The next part of the routine is a line, as indicated by dots in Figure 17. I call this the crest of the foot. Again you may work from beneath the little toe up to but not underneath the big toe.

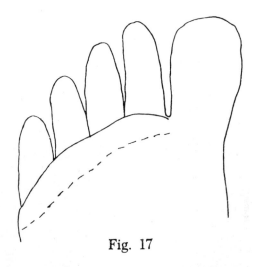

Fig. 17

At the base of each small toe, where it joins the top of the foot, are some important spots according to reports given on the work. When massaging just a spot, first locate the correct place by flexing the thumb joint and applying a light pressure until you are certain you have started cracking the crystals. Remember, not more than four times, or less than three on any given line or spot. This area of massage is visualized in Picture E.

53

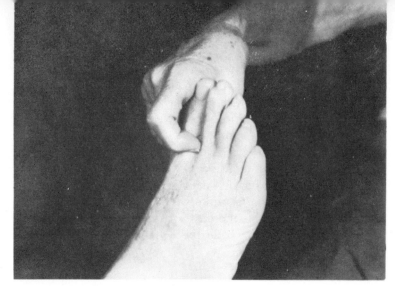

Picture E

Work on the other corner of the same toe will be indicated in Picture F.

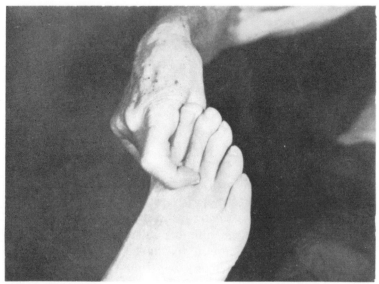

Picture F

Continue with a spot on each side of the other three toes, where they join the top of the foot and the toes are completed on the right foot.

Four lines are used for massage of the area, indicated as the back in Figures 4 and 6. Three of these lines will be marked by dots No. 1, No. 2, and No. 3 in Figure 18.

When working the line pointed out in Figure 18 by dots No. 2, some feet respond best by massaging from the heel up to the toe; others from the opposite direction. It seems that the crystals are snuggling under the bony structure of the foot. Therefore the thumb should be turned as if it might be trying to crawl up under the bones, and the crystalline deposits will crack more readily.

Lines vary in different feet as much as a quarter of an inch. Some rare person may feel nothing if you follow the very edge of the foot, as shown by dots No. 1 in Figure 18. If they feel nothing with the first trial, move up a little higher and try there. Sometimes they feel nothing in the foot, but if you move a small fraction of an inch and manipulate

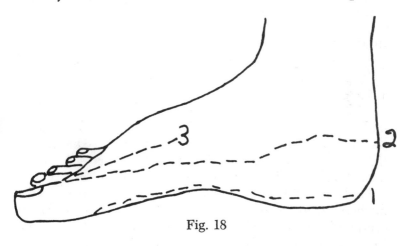

Fig. 18

along a line beside the other, they will writhe with pain.

The fourth line for the massage of the back area is shown

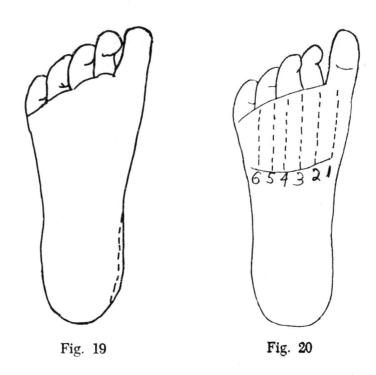

Fig. 19   Fig. 20

by the dots in Figure 19.

Six lines up across the ball of the foot are next in the routine. In Figure 20, they are marked by dots numbered 1, 2, 3, 4, 5 and 6.

These lines begin well up underneath the ball of the foot, and continue up toward but not on the line at the crest of the foot, as indicated by the dots in Figure 17. This part of the massage covers part of the thyroid, all the solar plexus, liver, lungs, and bronchial tubes, as marked in Figure 4.

Find the gall bladder as shown in Figure 4. Use the same method already described for isolated spots. Massage the ascending colon line as shown in Figure 4. You may need to go from the ileocecal valve up to the transverse colon, or the opposite. The ileocecal valve, being at the end of this line, receives its massage along with the ascending colon.

Massage the area for the transverse colon as designated in Figure 4.

Make two lines across the stomach and pancreas area, as shown by dots 1 and 2 in Figure 21. Begin each of these lines at the edge of the foot as the dots indicate, and move in toward the middle of the foot until the thumb doing the massage feels a tendon where these lines end.

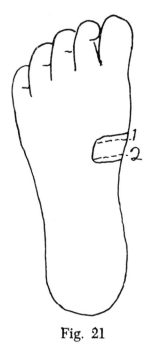

Fig. 21

Look at Figure 4 for the line marked kidney, with the adrenal gland at the top. Massage up or down this line as you find necessary on the foot with which you are dealing. If this is thoroughly accomplished, the adrenal gland will receive its massage along with the kidney.

Follow this with the line given as bladder and ureter tube in Figure 4. Next is the sciatic nerve, designated in Figure 4.

Find the spot pointed out as uterus or testicle in **Figure** 6. It is usually halfway between the anklebone and the point of the heel. However, sometimes it is a little backward or forward. Use the technique for single small areas.

Work around the anklebone on the circular line marked in Figure 6 as the lymph glands in the groin and armpits. To crack the crystals well you need at times to massage this with the thumbnail turned toward the anklebone. On another foot it may require exactly the opposite. I cannot stress too much the fact that you should not give up easily.

For the area of the rectum, as given in Figure 6, it may require either up or down massage. This line extends along the Achilles tendon upward, curving enough at the top of it to continue up the middle of the back of the leg to around seven inches from the bottom of the heel.

Find the line marked hand, elbow, and shoulder in **Figure** 7. Massage this up or down, as you find necessary. In **Figure** 4, find a line which is labeled "hand," "elbow," and "shoulder," and massage accordingly.

Look at Figure 7 for the curved line marked hip. On the human foot you can find that line by a joint of the bones halfway along the ouside of the foot from the little toe to the back of the heel. As indicated in Figure 7 by the curved line, half-circle that joint. As already instructed, on any line or spot work not less than three or more than four.

From this curved line work along the edge of the foot on the line marked "knee" and "foot" in Figure 7. Again, if you feel nothing when you are massaging in one direction, try it the other way. As marked "hip," "knee," and "foot" in Figure 4, massage that line.

In Figure 7, locate the spot designated as prostate or ovary. Follow previous instructions given for a single small area. Circle the ankle bone, as shown in Figure 7 to be the lymph glands in the groin and armpits. Follow the line shown as rectum in Figure 7, along the Achilles tendon, up to its top, where this joins the line of the rectum from the inside of the leg. Follow each of the two lines marked flat of the shoulders, and the two lines given for the breast as in Figure 7.

That completes the massage of the right foot, with the exception of what we call the "candy" because it simply feels good and is very relaxing. Begin by taking between your fingers one toe at a time. Rotate the toe four times to the left, and four times to the right, and pull gently as if you were trying to stretch the toe.

Notice I said "gently." I have seen some people grab the toe as if they thought it was about to escape them. They would twist vigorously and pull as if they intended to bring it out of its socket.

Such bear-like maneuvers spoil the entire relaxing effect. Now rotate the entire foot four times to the right, and four times to the left. Draw the foot slowly backward and forward. This completes the right foot.

Begin and continue on the left foot exactly the same as the right until you have completed the six lines up across the ball of the foot. Notice, in Figure 5 that the area marked "pancreas" extends completely across the foot. Accordingly you massage two lines across the bottom of the left foot.

Unless the foot is extremely long, such as a size fourteen, and the thumb of the masseuse is very small, these two lines across the foot will not only massage the stomach and pancreas but will also cover the transverse colon area. Go up or down, as needed, along the descending colon. Next, manipulate along the kidney line, as given in Figure 5. From this point on, the routine for the left foot is the same as the right.

If at this point you are thinking that this is too much and you can never get it, let me assure you that one masters the entire routine much sooner than you think, if you just study and follow directions.

I have seen beginners require more than two hours the first time for only the right foot. The second time they would do both the right and left in two hours. The third massage, they could complete both feet in one hour.

The usual time for the experienced to do this routine on an average pair of feet is forty-five minutes. On an extremely big foot, both of them may require an hour; on a child's feet it might be accomplished in thirty minutes or less.

If you are a rank amateur, do not be discouraged by the lengthy explanations. They were given in detail to save you the time which the author spent years in acquiring.

Chapter Five

ROUTINE FOR THE HANDS AND
EXPLANATION OF MANIPULATIONS

The routine for the hands is basically the same as for the feet. Begin on the thumb of the right hand, with three lines up the outside and then three up the inside. Continue with exactly the same routine for the thumb as the one given for the big toe.

The fingers are the same as was given for the smaller toes untill you reach the line called the crest of the foot. On the hand there is no room for two lines across beneath the fingers; therefore you do only one line from the little finger, around the base of each finger, and slightly in between, including the index finger.

Next are the spots on each side of every finger where it joins the back of the hand. This is done exactly the same as is brought out in Pictures D and E, which illustrate that work on the toes.

For the back area, do the lines as given by dots 1, 2 and 3 in Figure 22.

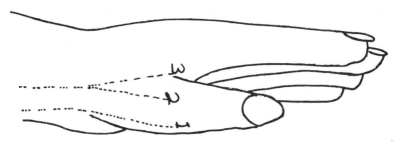

Fig. 22

As marked in Figure 8, continue with the thyroid, solar plexus, and liver, doing six lines up across the ball of the hand, the same as we did on the foot. Then the gallbladder, ascending colon, transverse colon and two lines across the stomach and pancreas area as shown in Figure 8. Next are the kidneys, ureter tube, bladder, sciatic nerve, uterus or testicles, as also indicated in Figure 8.

Unlike the routine for the foot I usually do the shoulder, elbow, hand, hip, knee, foot, and rectum in one long line as they are given in Figure 8. Then I turn the hand over and do another long line as the shoulder, elbow, hand, hip, knee, foot and rectum, marked in Figure 10.

This completes the right hand, with the exception of the "candy," which is given on the fingers and hand exactly the same as the toes and foot. The left hand is the same as the right, until the six lines up across the ball of the hand are completed.

After this, just as you crossed the left foot, you now work from the thumb to the outside of the hand as given in Figure 9, to be the stomach, pancreas, and transverse colon. Make one or two lines across, depending on the size of the hand being massaged and the breadth of the thumb performing the manipulations.

Next are the descending colon and the kidney, and from there the left hand is completed exactly as the right.

IMPORTANCE OF MANIPULATIONS

When I began this work I had only one manipulation, and I quit and despaired on some people because the crystals would not crack with that single movement. In Chapter Four, the explanation was made that going up a line instead of down or vice versa might be the difference between cracking or not breaking the crystals.

In the vast majority of feet the crystals are relatively easy to break and can be worked out with a very simple type of compression massage, so that will be given first.

Always be sure that your fingernails are as short as they can be filed without becoming sore. That will ensure the confidence in both the recipients and the masseuse that what they feel is from the cracking crystals and not from the fingernail of the thumb or finger used in the massage.

Since the ball of the thumb is soft, it is not effective in this work. Therefore turn the corner of the thumb down on the line being followed on the foot and move forward by flexing the thumb joint, as shown in Figure 23 by Motion 1 and Motion 2.

MOTIONS OF THUMB

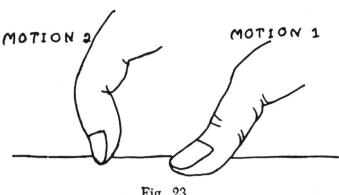

Fig. 23

Motion 1 and Motion 2, as illustrated in Figure 23, must be done consecutively and so close together on the line being followed that the thumb appears to be crawling by little nibbles. If Motion 1 and Motion 2 are further apart, many of the crystals will not be cracked and time and effort are wasted.

It requires patience and perseverance to acquire a nimble use of these movements. If continuous effort is made, the time will come when the thumb will fairly fly along the line on the foot.

Once I was massaging a man's feet when he asked, "Is this all you do all day long?" When I told him it was, he said, "My, you've got an easy job."

"Have you ever tried wiggling your thumb all day and half of the night?"

He looked at me for a minute, and then started to laugh. He had never thought of it in that light. *This* incident shows how nimble you can become with these manipulations if once you have really learned them. After that, you have the use of it for the rest of your life.

When I first started to do this massage professionally I would only do two or three pairs of feet in a day and my hands and arms would ache from weariness halfway to my elbows. After the work progressed, I did as many as twelve pairs of feet with no discomfort except general weariness.

Not only have my hands become accustomed to continual movement, but I have also discovered the easiest possible way to perform the manipulations. A beginner will use the entire hand in Motion 1 and Motion 2, and I have seen them involve the entire arm. That is so much wasted effort, because it is not even needed. Learn to flex only the joint in the middle of your thumb. Practice this until you can do it without strain. Then simply allow your hand to glide along with the thumb.

Another mistake the amateur invariably makes is that he thinks it must take lots of pressure to crack those crystals. In the average hand or foot, this not only is wrong but the extra force is even injurious to the tender little nerves to which the crystals are attached. The thumb must snuggle against the surface of the foot being massaged in order to follow the sharp little curves. However, it is the quick and dexterous turn of the thumb which performs the correct trick on the crystals and causes them to break.

Many people have said to me, "Your hands must be very strong."

If you are a masseuse, and doing foot massage professionally, all the strength required in your hands is to be able to keep the thumb or finger wiggling hour after hour. Invariably, when the crystals begin to disappear, the party being massaged will remark that I am not pushing as I was. The truth is that I was using very little pressure at first, but to them it felt as if I were coming down with a hundred pounds. That was caused by so many crystals pressing on and distressing the tiny nerves.

There are times when the forefinger, or the one next to it, will accomplish the work better than the thumb. Also, in this case, the corner of the finger, because it is firm and not the pad should be used — Picture G.

I have found quite a few feet which did not feel the simple massage just described except the light pressure of my thumb or finger. Bcause predecessors in this work had contended that if there was a problem in the body there were crystals in the feet, I was puzzled. Then the thought arose

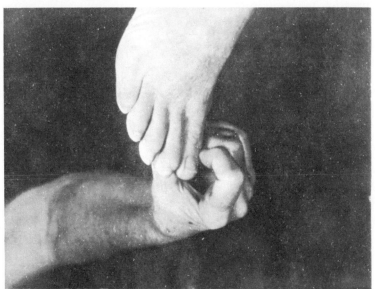

Picture G

that if they were correct, the crystals were there but were not being broken by this manipulation.

The determination followed that some method must be evolved to perform the work on these feet also. After perhaps months, or even a year or two (I kept no record of the time) I developed two new manipulations. It is outstanding to know that the feet on which these cracked the crystals did not respond to any other movement.

The first one of these manipulations I will explain I have named the "screwdriver" because of the similarity of the motion to the use of that tool.

Figure 24 illustrates this manipulation.

Turn the thumb as shown by Motion 1 in Figure 24, then Motion 2, Motion 1, and Motion 2, and on and on. Between each turn of the thumb allow it to move very slightly forward along the line being followed on the foot.

I have seen people, who felt nothing from the simple compression massage, almost writhe with pain when this movement was used. However, there were those who felt nothing

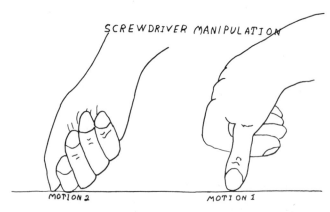

Fig. 24

with either the compression or the screwdriver manipulation, and that was when I developed what I call the "side-wind."

It is illustrated by Motion 1 and Motion 2 in Figure 25.

In Figure 25, notice that the thumb is turned one way but the line on the foot which is being followed runs the opposite direction. The thumb joint is flexed to make Motion 1 and Motion 2, but in between each of these the thumb glides very slightly sideways. It seems to be crawling in that direction while it's bending the other.

Since I have used these three manipulations and tried them forward and backward, and have also moved a little one way or the other from the line as found in the average

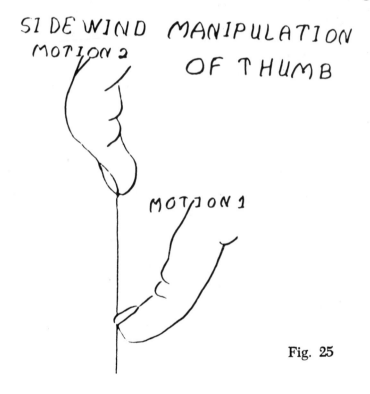

SIDE WIND MANIPULATION
MOTION 2
OF THUMB

MOTION 1

Fig. 25

foot, I have not failed to have those persons tell me they certainly felt more than my thumb and finger. Of course the people who call me always have problems in their bodies.

AFTER THE MASSAGE

Three months after every crystal is gone from a pair of feet, it is well to check them with a complete massage to find if any more crystalline deposits have formed. If not more than three complete routines are required to free them this time, then wait six months and try again. If after half a year they feel nothing in their feet, I forget about them. Entire families I have not seen for four or five years, but have talked with them by phone, tell me they are having no problems.

When I am giving compression twice a week, which is the best length of time between massages, I insist that they rub their feet on the days they are not coming to me. Their simple method of pressure will not perform what the manipulation I give would accomplish, but it will keep the broken crystals from settling back and growing.

Also, after the blood has dissolved the crystals and there is no further need for me to massage their feet, if they rub them four or five minutes each day it will help to keep the crystalline deposits from forming again.

One mother told me that she made it her daily chore to rub the feet of each member of her family. She said it was well worth it to have the assurance they were not going to be sick with something she might thus prevent. Quite a few women have told me they rub their feet when they have their bath because the feet are easy to massage when they are wet.

CHAPTER SIX

THE MOUTH, ESOPHAGUS, STOMACH AND INTESTINAL TRACT

In a chiropractor's office I saw a chart showing the pneumogastric nerve, commonly called the vagus nerve. It originates from the medulla oblongata which is that part of the brain situated between the cerebellum and the spinal cord. Actually the medulla appears to be a continuation of that cord.

This vagus nerve, as was illustrated on that chart, comes out of the medulla oblongata and continues down the neck with branches to the eyes, ears, nose, throat, lungs, heart, stomach, liver, and colon. More than one chiropractor has told me that this nerve can definitely be affected by pressures in the neck from slipped vertebrae.

Consider, therefore, how important is the care of the neck. Also remember this significance when massaging the neck area in the big toe. To realize this, look for the neck in Figure 4 and Figure 5.

More than one person has told me that their stomach ulcers had completely quit bothering them after their feet were cleared of crystals by these foot massages. A lady to whom I will refer as P. S. had heard some of the reports given by these people about their ulcers; she was really excited about having her feet massaged.

Before the work was begun with P. S. she told me to relieve her pain the vagus nerve had been severed from her stomach. Immediately I was reluctant to take her money. I explained to her that according to all I had read and seen on charts, the branches of the vagus nerve were the main controlling stimuli. She insisted on trying the foot massage. Because there were nerves from the spinal cord to the stomach, it seemed as if there might be a faint hope. The work was begun, and we continued for more than twenty routines. Unlike the others with ulcerated stomachs, she reported no improvement.

May I again emphasize that I am not a dietician and make no claims to be completely authentic on the subject of nutrition, but I would like to make a few observations which have been called to my attention.

Very few men would think of mistreating their cars the way they neglect and burden their poor stomachs either because of ignorance or extreme disregard. They would be too concerned financially if for no other reason. They may complain about their doctor bills, but fail to consider for one minute that daily they contribute to those expenses by what they do or do not put into their mouths.

The way food enters the mouth can also be of vast importance. The simple procedure of chewing is neglected by the best of us, yet what an important part it plays in the repair bills required by our bodies. If you do not believe me, I dare you to try this simple experiment. It can be quite enlightening.

It is more interesting if four or five people are seated about the table. A very hard coconut macaroon from the health store is quite good for this test. If it is so hard that you must use the point of a paring knife and a little wooden mallet with which to strike the handle in order to separate the macaroon into two equal parts, so much the beter. Explain that each person is to take half of a macaroon into his mouth. He is not to chew, but simply hold it in his mouth until all of it has gone down his throat in syrup except the coconut.

As each one puts his piece of macaroon into his mouth, drop half of one into a glass of water. There will be very little or no talking at first because every mouth will be too full. You will probably sit there looking at each other with amusement and feeling a little silly to have tried such a thing. But sit tight.

One by one they will report that all of the half of a macaroon is gone except the cocoanut. When the last one has swallowed the final drop of syrup into which his piece of small cake has been converted, then take the fragment from the glass of water and break it open. You will probably find it bone dry in the center. At least that is what we discovered when we tried this.

What does this prove? If we keep the food in our mouths long enough to allow the saliva to function, digestion does begin there. We should learn to chew and chew and chew. The hurry and flurry in the average American's life has no time for such minor details. He must swallow quickly in order to plunge ahead into the race to live in this society and consequently his poor duodenum must do what it can to digest the starch that has been tossed down into it.

I can just hear more than one saying, "What in the world has this to do with foot massage?"

Let me tell you quickly that it has everything in the world to do with foot massage. My work as a masseuse is definitely repair. According to Dr. Fitzgerald and Dr. Riley, you would not need me if you did not have crystls. When do the crystals come? When you have an injury to the body. When you do not chew, the duodenum has been insulted, and it is a definite part of the body. This is not all that is involved in the failure to chew.

The proteins are cast down into the stomach in chunks and left there for the discomfort of the poor hydrochloric acid in its struggle to digest that which has not been prepared for it. Then what happens?

"What in the world is the trouble with my stomach that I'm always belching?"

It may be that you cannot bring the gas up, and your middle feels like a big rock had settled on it. You must have something to lift the discomfort and so you take whatever happens to be in your purse or your pocket. Shortly you are happy again, and so you rush ahead in your mad race to live.

Your poor stomach is still nobly fighting down there to get the valve in the pyloric orifice open and throw this entire mess out into the duodenum. It knows from experience it must get it off of its hands before you toss it some more cake or pop or ice cream or whatever your long-perverted appetite happens to choose.

The valve in the pyloric orifice is stubborn to the last degree. It has not been properly considered. It is not supposed to open until the food has been thoroughly digested in the stomach, to say nothing of the correct amount of acid to wash against it and cause its spring to open its doors.

At last it either balks completely and throws you into the hospital for an operation, or it gives up and meekly opens its door saying, "Duodenum, don't blame me. This entire disagreeable concoction started further up the assembly line and there is nothing I can do about it. Here it is."

The duodenum has not recovered from the bad mood of yesterday's espisode, so does not try too hard. It just shoves it along into the jejunum and the ileum, where the blood and the lymph are supposed to pick up something of value for the body.

They find painfully little to grab, so they are also insulted, and the only thing left is to discard this mass into the colon if the ileocecal valve has not become disrupted by this time. Maybe it will open and maybe it will not. If it does not, we have constipation. Oh, well, it does not make much difference now. Putrefaction has already set in and given the blood a good healthy dose of poison acid. The blood thus loaded moves slowly, but that is nothing new. Your blood has always been lazy and required circulation pills for years.

The ileocecal valve did open, but the colon has been sore for years and shrunken in spots and bulged in others. What of it? You just rush down and get a colonic, and then you'll feel so clean. You sure will. You will be cleansed of all the friendly germs along with mucus which God created to lubricate the alimentary canal. Also this is a repair bill, just like the foot massage. If you had no problem, you would not be there.

Tell me the truth, now. Would you treat the motor of your car in that fashion? Of course you would not. It would be too expensive to keep it running. How about the cost of your alimentary canal? The doctor, the drugs, yes, and the foot massages to break the crystals you have just obtained. Don't forget, they have been forming for years in the feet of this nonchewing individual if it is true injury to the body that produces them.

You wonder why I should worry—since it all means more money for me. Of course I am a masseuse who rubs for the cash, but if I did not have a humanitarian spark in my heart I would not be worthy of the name. Also, who labors and does not desire success? I cannot attain results if you persistently build more crystals.

Go into a doctor's office and look at the load of sick, distressed people with whom he is pursued each day. He puts out literature, but who has time to read? I do hope you will read this, stop and consider, and start chewing.

Maybe you are certain you already chew thoroughly. Is your dry food a liquid when it leaves your mouth? It should be. Many years ago they advocated chewing each mouthful fifty times before swallowing.

Figure 26 is a chart of the alimentary canal as our old physiologies described it. Remember that this is a diagram and not a picture, so please do not confuse it with its actual appearance.

One woman who was suffering the discomforts of a hernial diaphragm reported that after the foot massages it had entirely quit bothering her. Another who had the same problem told me that she was much relieved after several routines on her feet. She was quite pleased with the improvement,

73

DIAGRAM OF ALIMENTARY CANAL

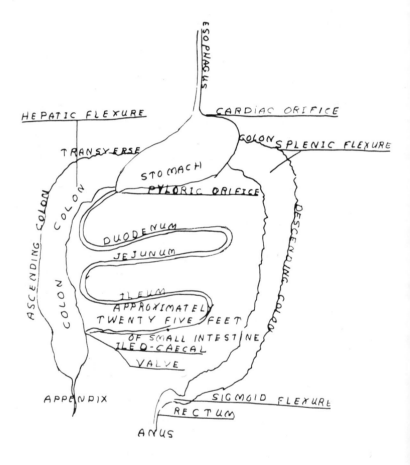

Fig. 26

because her doctor had said that a large portion of her stomach was pushed up through the opening in the diaphragm.

When I gave her the first foot massage, A. R. told me that for five years her bowels had not moved without the assistance of an enema and for twenty-five years had not moved for as long as a week without the same help. I assured her that we were going to work to get her to experience an evacuation twice a day without any help.

She said, "Woman, that will be the day."

Three months after all crystals seemed to be gone from her feet, she called me to tell me that, "the day" had come. Action had been normal twice a day with no prompting help of any sort, and once a day for some time, but she would not call me until she had reached the goal I had set for her.

I find many people who express surprise at the idea of the necessity for more than once-a-day evacuation. When my youngest son was less than five years of age, I was puzzled because his movements were regularly three times a day. I told our family doctor, who assured me that this was normal and something to be desired by everyone. One day, at seven in the morning, my son accidentally swallowed a safety pin.

As any mother would be, I was terribly alarmed and called the doctor for help. He told me not to do anything but just wait and watch. At seven the next morning the pin came through him. The doctor assured me that my son was one child whose alimentary canal was functioning on schedule.

Many people have asked me if it is possible for these foot massages to stop constipation. They invariably tell me they have asked because they had such a marked improvement along that line.

When I went to give one woman her third foot massage she met me at the door, laughing and said, "If I knew you did to me what I strongly suspect you did, I don't know if I'd allow you to touch me again or not."

Two nights after I had given her the regular foot routine

she started cramping in a fashion similar to a diarrhea pain and hurried to the bathroom. The feces were not loose, as she had feared from the feelings she had developed, but normal except that there was a huge amount.

All night it seemed as if she was hardly back in bed when she must again rush to the bathroom. The next morning it continued. She wondered if she might have intestinal flu, but no aches or pains accompanied this disorder. Then as suddenly as it had begun, it stopped; and her description was that she had never felt more wonderful in her life.

A very small minority have had their elimination stop completely after the foot massages, and nothing but a good enema could change the situation. About half a dozen out of more than a thousand have reported this reaction.

One woman had suffered for fifty years from hemorrhoids even though she had undergone an operation for them when she was young. Seven years ago she was given these routines on her feet, and reports that she has had no such problem since. Others say they have been able to avoid an operation since the massage on their feet.

A little boy of five had suffered much from a problem with his bowel movements. His mother said it was pitiful to see him want so badly to eliminate when nothing came. The doctors could find no reason for his trouble. The only comfort they could give the parents was he would probably outgrow the condition.

They were visiting his mother's parents when her father was being given the massages. They could only be there for two routines on the little boy's feet, but they felt it was worth a try. Later the family told me that two times did the job because by the time they reached home their son's problem had ceased. That was six years ago, and they have reported it had never returned.

Another young boy was embarrassed because he would not know he had eliminated until he found it in his clothing. It seemed to be an inherited weakness of some sort, because his father and his paternal grandfather had experienced the same situation in their younger days.

The doctors could give the mother no reason or solution. As in the other case, they thought perhaps he would grow out of his difficulty. In the meantime the mother and her son were quite distressed by his situation. This boy was given a dozen foot massages and the progress, if any, was slow and very little evidence of any improvement. At last, some time after the crystals were gone from his feet, his mother reported that his trouble had ceased.

Chapter Seven

THE BRAIN AND THE NERVES

It is a generally accepted fact that massage of any kind is soothing and helpful to the nerves. However, I am convinced that where the nerve cell itself is damaged, very little if anything will be accomplished by the foot massage.

Some case histories wil be given here to illustrate situations to which I am referring. My experience with foot massage and Parkinson's disease has been with two men and one woman. Each told me it was caused by a dead brain cell, according to the explanation of the doctors. One man told me that his doctor advised surgery. Each of these people thoroughly tested out the foot massage. They did report some improvement in other areas, but felt no benefit for the Parkinson's.

Two women, at various times and in different locations who were suffering from multiple sclerosis, called for me to massage their feet. One of them told me that her doctor had said it was a deterioration of the sheathe or outside covering of the nerve which had brought about her condition. Both women went on and on with the massages. Being desperate, they hated to give up in despair. One even continued until twenty-five routines had been done on her feet. It was all to no avail. Neither woman felt any definite improvement.

I have also found that a tumor on the nerve itself gives no response to foot massage. I have had experience with one man and two women, each of which had a tumor on a nerve in the foot. Work on the hands was tried, but no results were reported. The tumors continued to grow until removed by surgery.

One woman said that the night after I gave her the routine on her feet, a small tumor on her ankle pained her a great deal. It had been there for several months, and she had asked her doctor to remove it. He refused, because he feared that her ankle might become stiff. The second night after the foot massage she experienced pain in the same tumor again.

She told her husband, "I'm not going to let that woman touch me again. She's done something to that tumor." The morning efter the second night she called to her husband, "That woman sure has done something to that tumor. The pain's gone, and the tumor is gone." You can be assured that she continued until she felt nothing but my thumb and finger going over her feet.

An elderly lady in her eighties had a tumor on the bottom of her foot. It did not pain her unless she stepped down on it, but the location of it made walking almost impossible unless pressure was put on it. It was as big around as a silver half-dollar and protruded all of half an inch. After eight foot massages she told me she could not even feel where it had been when she rubbed her fingers over the spot.

A young girl of fifteen had a tumor on her neck. The doctor told her parents he did not know what type it was. He thought they should operate and make tests to find out the nature of it. The parents and the girl wanted to try the foot massages first.

After the fifth routine on her feet, her mother told me that the tumor had shrunk to half of its former size; and when her feet were completely cleared of the crystals, the mother said it was entirely gone. Three or four years later they reported to me that it had not returned.

One man was introduced to me by some of his friends, who said he had brain damage which had bothered him from birth. He was a fine-looking man in his late forties and handled himself so well that his problem was not easily detected. His friends said that his biggest symptom, which they noticed, was that he could not switch subjects quickly when in a conversation. If you changed, he would just sit there and stare.

He described some of his problems to me. He drove a car, and had a job in an airplane factory. One day, uptown in Phoenix, he came out of a business office and could not remember where he had parked his car. That was not so unusual; but he could not remember what make it was, or how it looked. He stood there on the street for thirty minutes before he could recall the appearance of his car. Another day he got into his car, and for twenty minutes could not remember how to start it.

He said it could at times be a most distressing thing with which to cope, and he wanted to try the foot massages. It required eighteen routines to clear his feet of the crystals. That was five years ago, and his friends tell me he has been most alert ever since the work on his feet. They say he can and often does switch subjects in a conversation with them just to prove to himself that he can. He told me he no longer had loss of memory and he considered the money he had paid me the best-spent cash in his life.

I was called to work on the feet of an elderly man who had suffered a stroke. He had no use of one arm and one leg and his speech was labored and scarcely intelligible. His wife explained that she did not expect me to help him. She had only called me because he felt that nothing was being done for him, and this would pacify him.

When I did the work, he would lie on the bed. I would sit at the foot of the bed and spread a towel under his feet because I used a little light oil to make my hands glide easily. As he could not move one foot, I always picked it up and placed it on the towel. The third massage, when I started to reach for his paralyzed foot to put it on the towel, he moved it over himself. He smiled at my surprise.

When I was giving him the fifth routine on his feet he

showed me how he could draw the paralyzed knee up to his chest and lift the hitherto useless foot straight up into the air.

He looked so happy; but his wife called me into another room and told me again that she did not expect me to do anything for him. But the day before he had walked across the street and visited with a neighbor for an hour, and he had done nothing like that since his stroke. He could now speak some words quite distinctly. In short, she was dismissing me because he was improving.

When I closed the door behind me I heard the poor old fellow pleading, "Please, have her come back. Please." I certainly would have been glad to go back and find out exactly how much recovery of the use of his body he would report to me.

Once I was called to give these massages to a young married woman who had suffered problems all her life with her nerves and was at that time struggling against a complete collapse. She had been treated in a very reputable psychiatric hospital, but her husband said she was growing steadily worse.

I do not remember the exact number of routines done on her feet, but I do know it was several. A few weeks after they were finished, her husband told me she was one hundred percent better.

For years a business man had suffered from what the doctors called "nerve fatigue". He was taking pain pills, tranquilizers, and sleeping tablets. Both he and his wife described his condition as growing steadily worse. As a last hope, he decided to try the foot massages. After each routine he would be so dizzy he could not stand or walk alone and both feet would be completely numb and feel as if they were not there. After the eleventh massage he said he was not dizzy, his feet were not the least bit numb, and he felt nothing but my thumb and fingers going over his feet.

Three months later, I called him to tell him we should massage his feet and see if any crystals had come back. "Oh,

81

Ina," he said, "I'm feeling just fine. Besides that I'm too busy." I tried to tell him he should find out about the crystals before he had pain, but he would not hear me.

Eight or nine months later he called me and had me come right then. All his old aches and pains had returned with their former force. Something like six more routines, and his feet were again cleared of the crystalline deposits.

When I called him after three months, he told me to come right over. That time it required about three massages. Six months after that, four or five complete routines again cleared the crystals from his feet. Then the day came that, after six months, he still felt nothing but my thumb and fingers massaging his feet lightly.

Elsewhere in this book I have made the statement if they have no crystals after six months have elapsed, I forget about them. All this happened six years ago. A short time ago I talked with this man, and he told me that since I had seen him he had taken no drugs and had not experienced any physical difficulty.

I could go on and on giving similar examples, but these should suffice. On those whose nerves were easily disturbed I have given Swedish on the head, neck, shoulders, and back. Gradually both the recipients and I realized that something more than Swedish was being done.

I often strayed from the true manipulations of the Swedish to some movements of my own, which seemed to give the highly excited nerves a feeling of tranquility. As I would drag my second finger from the thumb on the right hand across the head or shoulder which I was massaging, there would be intermittently a light popping or cracking sound. It was similar to that produced by walking across a nylon rug and then touching a metal door knob.

Those who want to dispose of the idea quickly and easily say it is my finger joint snapping. I definitely know that it is not. I can even feel the light pop at the end of my finger in the flesh just beneath the skin of the person being massaged.

A woman on whose head I had often done the "popping" massage, as it has been called, was given a brainwave test. For three days after the brain wave I could not make the cracking sound on the skull area of her head, although I tried repeatedly. At the very same time the "popping" massage worked as usual on her neck and shoulders.

Another peculiar circumstance is that I can only produce this sound with one finger of each hand. I can rub either thumb or any other finger across flesh in exactly the same fashion and position and there will be no sound.

One woman, who was greedy for this type of massage, paid me five dollars to do this on her neck and shoulders for an hour. I then realized that for me to continue this too long in succession caused the snapping to become fainter and fainter, and my finger became terribly weary. Also I have found a reasonable amount to be as effective as twice that much.

People with injured joints say they have found nothing to equal its use on the damaged articulation. One man had an injured knee from his service in the army. Even though it happened more than twenty years ago, the joint would become so swollen and painful he could hardly force himself to use it. If he carried a heavy load, which often became necessary in his work, it would sometimes completely give away and allow him to go down.

He asked me to try this snapping massage on the knee. He said that just as we heard the sound it was as if a hot electrical needle had darted right through the middle of the joint. His wife had experienced the same manipulation on some of her arthritic joints and told me it was like something hot going through where the bones met, but I had thought that perhaps she felt it because of her arthritis. The man told me that almost immediately the swelling began to subside, and the pain and stiffness to disappear.

83

I wondered if the relief really came from that or if it might be that the massage on the feet had brought about improvement by way of the nerves, and the snapping massage was merely a pacifier while the slower method, by way of the nerves zones, was working. Later something happened which clarified my decision on that.

This man's feet were clear of crystals and his knee was good with one exception. Across the kneejoint, at the top and just above the kneecap, there remained a swelling which stiffened the joint and made walking not quite normal. We both remembered I had never circled the kneecap with the popping massage.

After the second application of this massage around the kneecap he said, "No one can make me believe it is anything but this peculiar popping massage has done the job with this knee. The swelling is gone, along with every symptom of pain, and I have been carrying heavy loads every day this week."

Another man had an elbow which had been crushed when he was a young man. He had heard about the popping massage, and we tried it on his injured joint. He vowed it gave him almost immediate relief. He did not feel any hot electrical-needle effect as had the other man.

A woman who had been given the compression massage on her feet had a knee which was swollen and painful. After six of the popping massages around the joint she said the swelling and pain were entirely gone. As the work was being done on her knee, she said she also felt as if a hot needle ran straight into where the bones joined.

I wish I knew more about this, because a multitude of people claim there is nothing quite like it. I cannot believe I am the only one who has this gift; although I have tried to show a hundred people how to do it, but they could not create the sound or the effect.

Something I read about magnetic healing made me wonder if this was not connected with magnetic electricity. The article said that very few people had the gift and were not aware of it. They simply staggered on the fact that they had something and the method of using it.

When you read this, try it. Do not try just once, but again and again. One day I just realized I had something people thought was very valuable to them.

In Picture H you will see my finger doing the popping massage on or rather around the man's kneecap. Picture I illustrates this on the shoulders.

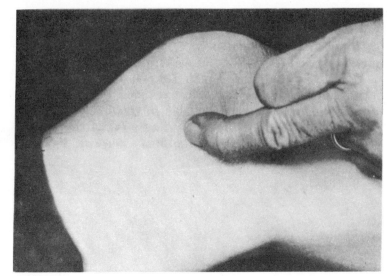

Picture H

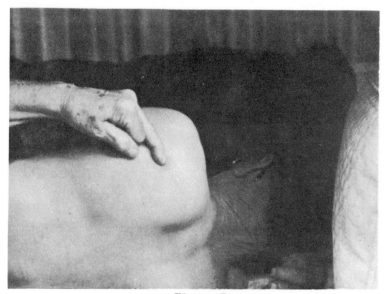

Picture I

CHAPTER EIGHT

THE HEAD, NECK, BACK, EARS, EYES, NOSE, AND THROAT

One woman had a whiplash neck injury. For eleven years she had been the victim of horrible headaches. She bought aspirins in the largest bottles and practically ate them all day. When the pain could not be curbed to be endurable, the doctor prescribed codine. For two years, every week she was given adjustments by a chiropractor. That gave her relief, but the next week the pain was there again as bad as ever.

When she was told about this work, she was ready to begin. Later, she told me she never did take another codine and only two aspirins after the first foot massage. It required fourteen complete routines on her feet to rid them of crystals. Being new in the work, and unaware that I should check her feet in three months, I did not contact her. It was eight months before she called me to come to her again.

The second time her feet were cleared in half a dozen massages. Half a year later she was given six more. We continued giving her the foot massages twice a year for two or three years. At last the day came when, after six months, she felt no crystalline deposits in her feet. She had developed the habit of rubbing her feet every day.

She told me that not only had her headaches gone long ago, but another wonderful thing had taken place in her body. For a number of years she had suffered with an ulcer at the entrance of the cervix. It had been treated by a doctor, who had carefully watched it for malignancy, but it semed as if there would never be any change.

After the crystals were out of her feet and had not returned for six months, her doctor told her, after one of her regular examinations that her ulcer was completely healed. She gave the complete credit to the foot massages. After five or six years, neither the headaches nor the ulcer had returned.

Another woman had severe headaches, and although she used nose spray constantly she could never breathe through her nostrils. She had such a pinched feeling in her throat that she sat up at night, with four pillows behind her, because if she should lie down she could not get her breath. When she first heard about the foot massages she was ready to try them. She told me that the doctors had given her tests and she was allergic to everything in her house and yard.

After the third routine on her feet, the next day such a headache hit her that she thought surely her head would burst and blow into bits. Just as she had decided she could not endure it another minute, as suddenly as it had begun it stopped, and that was the last of her terrible headaches. She still lives in the same house, and says she uses no nose spray and sleeps with one pillow under her head.

One woman told me that the foot massages had not lessened her headaches in the least; but six months after all crystals were out of her feet, she called me to say that her headaches had entirely disappeared.

One man had suffered for four years with a pain in his neck and down his back, in one arm and the corresponding leg. For six months his family pleaded with him to try the foot massages. At last he heeded, and the mainpulations were tried. On the third routine he felt nothing but the light pressure of my thumb and fingers. He said his pain was entirely gone. Four years later I called him just to inquire how he had been. "Couldn't be better," he assured me.

A woman whom the doctors had told had a ruptured disk in her back, decided she would try the foot massages. The first day I was there she showed me the back brace she was forced to wear. When she arose from a chair, she came up by hitches. She said the pain was too excruciating to describe. The doctors had told her that if they operated, her back would be stiff. When I had been over her feet the seventh time I asked if her back had improved.

"No," she told me. "If anything has changed, I would say it is worse."

When I gave her the ninth routine on her feet she happily announced she had danced the rhumba three nights in a row. On the eleventh massage, all crystals were gone from her feet. Later she said she had accomplished some very fancy steps in a dance festival and played volley ball in a tournament for four hours. She had given her back brace away.

A man and his wife, who had a baby eight months of age, were quite concerned about it. Every month of its life it had hard coughing and strangling spells. The doctor would give it penicillin and they would keep it under a vaporizer for four or five days. It would improve, but the next month the very same condition would return.

The mother told me that she had wanted to try the foot massages on the baby but had not because her husband had publicly ridiculed the entire idea. He was certain that people who claimed to be helped were not sick in the first place. They only thought they were sick and they believed these massages would help so they did.

One day the mother decided she was going to run the risk of taking things into her own hands and discover what the results would be. She brought the baby to me and asked me to massage his feet. As I did the manipulations, he fretted and at times cried out, indicating he felt discomfort.

Later the mother told me that all coughing stopped within an hour and a half after the routine was completed. She also said she was amazed to find the next stool passed after the foot massage was white and bubbly instead of the normal yellow. That had been the exact effect of the penicillin shot in the next bowel movement. The third foot massage, and the baby acted as if he felt nothing. So the work was stopped.

A few years later the mother told me that the baby never suffered another attack, and that the father was a firm believer in this work. She said he even made a point of telling people, before whom he had previously ridiculed foot massage, there was something to this thing after all. His baby did not think he was sick and did not even know what I was doing.

The case of another baby stands out in my mind. He was ten months old and could not sit up. He could not hold his head up any better than a newborn child. If you took hold of his hands, he would not pull as any normal infant would. If you pulled him up, he would hang and swing about like a limp sack.

The doctor had X-rayed his neck and back and found nothing wrong. He sent the child to a neurologist, who X-rayed his brain and gave it a brain wave test. He could find no damage there. In desperation they called me. They could not have been very hopeful when I began, because they continued to keep the baby in a bassinet.

The mother told me it almost jumped out of the basket before they knew it was moving. She heard its bottle fall to the floor. She ran in there because it had never thrown anything. She found it on its knees with its hands on the edge of the bassinet. She said that in another second it would have leaped out. She took it to the living room and laid it on the floor. It raised up on to its hands and knees and started making little jumps.

That child is now more than eight years of age, and just the past week its grandfather told me it was as lively and healthy as any of its brothers and sisters and was doing quite well in school.

An elderly man told me he had a peculiar experience. He had me to give him the foot massages because he had a pain in his shoulder. After I began the manipulations, the misery left his shoulder and went into the corresponding hip. It was so severe that he was confined to the bed.

However, he insisted that I continue with the routines on his feet. Next, a pain hit him in the lower back. At this time he was eighty-three years of age, and he told me that seventy years before a cow had kicked him backward and his back had hit a wagon tongue in the very same spot where the pain was now. For three weeks he was in bed while I continued to massage his feet. He said that slowly but surely all pain had left his shoulder, hip, and back, and at last he walked again with absolutely no discomfort.

I was called to work on the feet of a woman who was subject to unconscious periods of time which would continue as long as eight hours. The problem had begun shortly after she had stepped on a stone, turned her ankle, and fallen backward. These attacks would come as often as three or four times a week. She lost her job, and spent the small amount of money she had on the doctors. At last she was forced to see the county doctors, and the day came when they told her there was nothing more they could do.

I was told by the party who cared for this woman that she never had but one of those unconscious spells after the first massage on her feet.

When I began this massage I was told by a man, who had been doing the compression manipulations professionally for six years, what he did when someone had what he called "the shakes." He was not speaking of palsy but rather a loss of nerve control. He told me to massage the coccyx area of the foot. You will find this in Figure 27.

A woman, whom the doctors had told that she had heart and nerve attacks, came to me. She was thirty-three and had suffered from this trouble since she was fourteen. When I was doing the third routine on her feet, she quite suddenly began to gasp for breath and was shaking all over her body.

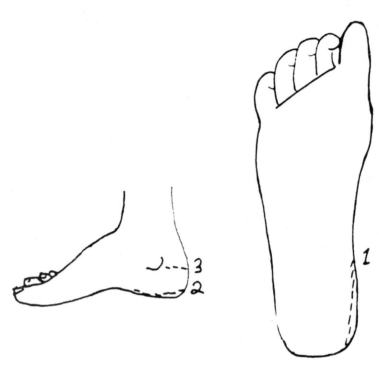

Fig. 27

In Chapter Eleven I will tell you what I did first, after which she quit gasping but was still shaking.

Second, I massaged the coccyx area on her foot as designated in Figure 27. Immediately she became quiet. Her husband, who was sitting by, told me he had watched the clock and just three minutes from the time she began to gasp and shake she was completely quiet. He also said that this never happened when she had one of these spells.

If he could not get her to a doctor, she would shake and gasp for her breath for an hour. If he did get her to the doctor, the physician would give her a shot which caused her to become limp and as if she were in a sort of stupor from which she would be two or three days recovering.

It required fourteen massages before the crystalline deposits were all gone from her feet. Five years later, a member of her family reported she had had no more heart and nerve attacks.

This woman's husband brought his mother to me. She was sixty-eight years of age. Twenty years before, she had been thrown from a truck and one of its wheels had passed over her at the waistline. They had thought she was dead at the time.

Since that accident, she had lived in a nightmare of suffering. She had dizzy spells which lasted for as long as eight hours, and so severe she would go into a cold clammy sweat. Her husband said he had spent hundreds of dollars on doctors and medicine, and did not know which way to turn for help. She was praying to die. Her son told me that when she was having those dizzy spells her eyes would twist until it looked as if they would almost come out of their sockets.

I gave her the first foot massage on a Monday. On Tuesday following they called me down to her house because she was going into one of those dizzy attacks. No one had told me what to do in a case like this, and I certainly prayed to God for wisdom. I massaged the entire back and neck areas on her feet (as shown in Figures 4, 5, and 6). Then I did some Swedish on her head and neck. Her son told me it was just ten minutes from the time I walked into the house until her dizziness was all gone.

The eighth foot massage she felt no crystals in her feet. Three months later she had two more routines on her feet and again felt nothing but my thumb and fingers. Six years afterward, I happened to meet her. Her eyes were bright, and her voice animated. She told me she had not felt even a twinge of the old dizziness.

Many times I have seen people shaking from uncontrolled nerves, and to massage the coccyx brought their assurance that the shaking was gone.

There are always exceptions, and one happened. The wife of a man to whom I had given four or five foot massages called and asked me to come at once. She said he was in bed and shaking all over. I massaged the coccyx areas on his feet, but, if anything, he only shook worse. I had to do something quickly. He needed help sooner than we could get him to his doctor, or get his doctor there.

I quickly thought that perhaps the upward slightly digging massaging, which I had given to various parts of the backbone of other persons, might work on this coccyx bone in his back. I tried it, and in a matter of seconds he told us the shaky feelings were gone. He says he has never had a spell like it since that time. Once he thought he was going to have it again; but by the time his wife called me and I got there, the sensation had passed.

From then on, if I found anyone with sharp crystals in the coccyx area on the foot, I showed a member of their family how to massage the last vertebra in the back.

A young college man whose feet I had massaged had quite sharp crystals in the coccyx. I showed his mother the manipulations I had used on the coccyx bone. He told me that when he started shaking when he was in school, he hurried to the rest room and worked around his coccyx bone himself. He said it immediately relieved him.

One time a man told me he had a constant and most annoying pain in his leg. I massaged his arm, and almost immediately he said the pain was gone. He was ready to believe that this was an exciting and miraculous thing. I told him I hated to disillusion him, but I had no desire to capitalize on something I knew was nothing but relief.

All that had been done was to divide the attention of the nerves between the lower and the upper part of the same nerve zone. This was also all I had done when I massaged the coccyx bone. It is wonderful to get relief at the time, but no one should feel that it dissolves his problem.

Neither is it a new thing. Our grandparents pinched one

part of the body to attract the attention of the nerves while they were doing something unpleasant to another area. Paul von Boeckman, in his course in psychiatry, told how to take pain out of a nerve center. He said snap the finger sharply but lightly striking the skin above the flesh right over the nerve center. That also works quite well.

Figure 28 demonstrates the drawing of pain away from the calf of the leg. Remember, in doing this that the point of the elbow corresponds to the kneecap, the shoulder to the hip joint, and the back of the hand to the top of the foot. This makes the calf of the leg analogous to the forearm on the same side as the palm of the hand.

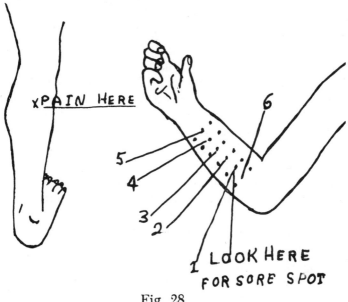

Fig. 28

As shown in Figure 28, find the first sore spot in the fore-arm. When you have located it with a little pressure by your thumb or finger, then massage lightly with a circular motion. Sometimes you will feel under your thumb a small bump

95

which will disappear as you continue to rub. After this light massage on that place for perhaps twenty seconds, look for another sore spot, as indicated by line and dot number 2 in Figure 28. When you have found it, repeat the light rubbing around and around over this place.

Continue with this as shown by lines and dots 3 and 4. Now drop back and see if you can find a sore spot that corresponds to line and dot 5. It is quite likely that you can find a row of sore spots up and down the forearm on either side of the first line. When there is a pain in the calf of the leg, I have found them even up to the shoulder. Usually they will end at the elbow.

As previously stated, this merely relieves the pain; but sometimes the discomfort is all the party having it can think about in that particular minute. Later you may be able to have a talk with the individual about the origin of his problem. Chiropractors may tell him it is from the pressure of a vertebra on a nerve in his back. The person whose life study is nutrition, will probably insist it comes from what he is or is not eating. One man who was suffering in this fashion said that the doctor told him it was his nerve ends. Another was told that all his pain came from his emotions.

One man who came to me said he had suffered with an aching in his leg until he was frantic. His wife said he had taken pain pills until he did not even act like himself. They both told me he had been in every one of the biggest clinics in the United States. In utter desperation, he had turned to the foot massage.

After sixteen routines, he said all the pain was gone, and for the first time in four years he was sleeping. Since there was no discomfort, he was going to discontinue the foot massage. I insisted that he might be sorry if he quit before he felt nothing but my thumb and finger, but he refused to listen.

Two months later he contacted me and had to have the manipulations on his feet at once because his pain had returned with fury. That time he continued until he felt no crystals cracking. A year later he told me the pain had not returned.

Something like thirty years ago, my neck was almost broken in an accident. The old country doctor did nothing but look at me and ask what had happened. There were no collars for that condition then, so you lived if you could. For a year I was unable to turn my head without taking my hands to push it to one side or the other. When at last it moved in a normal fashion, everyone thought it was all right and the accident was forgotten.

A year later, when my head began to shake, no one connected it with the accident. In Phoenix I met a chiropractor who told me that the palsy would go all over my body, and she was correct.

After it did, I began to have such dizzy spells two and three times a day that I would almost lose consciousness. The doctor wanted to give me tranquilizers, but I could not bear the thought of resorting to them. It was then that I heard about the classes of Eunice Ingham and I went to Dallas, Taxas, to hear her. I was so sick I actually wondered if I would live to return home. I did come back, and at once began to massage my feet.

Three or four months later I met an old friend. After I told her what I was doing she said, "Just looking at you would make a believer of me. The last time I saw you, you were shaking from head to foot. Now you do not even seem to have a tiny tremor. I can hardly believe my own eyes."

I was called to massage the feet of a man who had Bell palsy. He had been afflicted with it for twenty-five years. He told me he had not been able to close one eye for all those years except to take his fingers and pull the lid down, and then the minute he released it the eyelid would fly open.

He said that anyone who had not experienced such a thing could not possibly imagine the torture of never being able to close your eye. The eye ball was always so dry that the least movement was quite painful. His mouth was drawn down at one corner.

The fifth routine, he said, "Look! I can close my eye normally. It is an absolute miracle."

After the foot massages, one lady told me that her eyes were getting so bad she was worried about her vision. She went to her eye specialist. He gave her the necessary tests, and laughed at her fears. He told her that her vision was much improved but her glasses were not, and that was her problem.

Another woman had been informed she must have an operation for cataracts. She called me to massage her feet because of another physical disability. When she went in for the last examination before she was to have the cataracts removed, the doctor informed her that her eyes were so improved that he would not operate.

Another party told me she suffered with her neck, back, and eyes, but her eyes were the worst. She often walked the floor at night for as long as two hours because the pain was so severe she could not lie still. After eighteen foot massages, she reported that all her suffering was ended. Two or three years later, she told me it had not returned. I could go on and on with report after report.

CHAPTER NINE

THE GLANDS

The pituitary is said to be the most important or king gland in the body because it keeps all of the other glands functioning. It is no bigger than a cherry, and is suspended under the brain. I have been told by professional people that it is responsible for the growth or lack of development of the body. It also keeps the walls of the blood vessels healthy as well as regulating the speed of the heartbeats.

The parents of a boy of sixteen called me to massage his feet because he was so small and undeveloped. He resented the mere mention of his size because he was daily embarrassed about it. He was not even five feet tall, and his fourteen-year-old sister was five feet and eight inches. He drove a car, and was frequently stopped by the police who would look at his license and at him with a puzzled expression.

One highway patrolman said, "I'll have to let you go, but I still don't believe you're that old."

Faithfully the doctor had given him hormone shots for a year, hoping that they would assist his growth. There was not even a hint of fuzz on his face, and his voice was that of a child. After all those shots he was weighed and measured, and there was not even the tiniest fraction of a change.

On November Sixteenth he was given the first foot massage. He grumbled about it being silly, but his mother was determined that he was going to give it a thorough trial. On December Thirty-first, his mother measured him and told me he had grown a full inch and a half.

From that minute there was no more grumbling from this

boy. He would leave a ball game and come running if he saw my car approaching. His parents told me that in the next fifteen months he grew to five feet, eight and a half inches. He no longer shrank from standing beside his sister, but enjoyed the fact he was at least half an inch taller than she.

The sister had her problem. She was growing too fast to suit herself, and she was constantly annoyed by nose-bleed. Very shortly she was added to my list for foot massages. She had a doctor's permit to be excused from the physical education class because any little extra exertion caused her to hemorrhage from the nostrils.

The mother told me that her daughter also responded quickly. She said the nosebleed stopped almost immediately and the girl was happy to again be in the physical education class with her friends. Since that time, I have been told she did not grow any more.

The mother began to talk about her own problem. She was a beautiful woman but was being disfigured with what the doctors called wrong distribution of pigment in the skin. She had big splotches of white-looking skin with deep brown surrounding that. Some spots were developing on her face as well as on her body.

She had been told that the pituitary had some control over that condition also. Since her son and daughter had responded so well, she wanted the routine done on her feet.

I have no explanation for what happened in her case. She said that the white places on her skin immediately stopped spreading. A year or two later she told me that the white places had completely left her face, but not her body. She was not using anything on her face that had not been put on it before the foot massages.

Another boy of seventeen was very much under normal height. His father was five feet and six inches, and his mother five feet and two inches. Both the father and the son were so afraid he was going to remain extremely short that he was given the foot massages. The last I heard about him, he was a head taller than his father.

I have found that those who have bad headaches or severe cases of insomnia always have sharp crystals in the pituitary area. However, not everyone who has many crystalline deposits in the pituitary spot suffers from pain in the head or sleeplessness.

In writings and various ways the information has been made public which shows that if the walls of the blood vessels shrink causing the pressure to increase enough to force the blood through the smaller tubes, then the individual will register high blood pressure. The opposite can be true, and the walls so relaxed that consequently they bring the blood pressure low.

A man in his sixties passed out at work, and the attending nurse reported that his blood pressure was two hundred and thirty. He was taken home, and his natureopathic physician was called. He gave him herbs to lower his blood pressure. Three hours later, it was one hundred and ninety. The man asked his wife to call for me.

He was too sick to think of a complete foot massage, so I gave only the manipulation on the pituitary area of each big toe (shown in Figures 4 and 5). Three hours later, the naturopath again took his blood pressure. He expressed surprise and joy because it was then one hundred fifty over eighty.

THYROID

The thyroid gland consists of two lobes, each about two inches in length, which are connected by an isthmus. The lobes lie along each side of the larynx and upper trachea. They consist of a multitude of spaces filled with thyroxin which controls metabolism and growth. In case of a goiter, both sides or either one may become enlarged. It may be a cyst, or might be fibrous.

101

More than one person has told me after the foot massages that they were forced to cut down on medicine they were taking for the thyroid because they began to suffer from the symptoms of too much medicine. They said they felt that their gland was functioning better.

PARATHYROID

These glands are situated, one on each corner, in the two thyroid lobes. Their chief duty in the body is to control the distribution of calcium. In Chapter One is the account of the man with the calcified seventh cervical.

The foot massages were given to a woman who was afflicted with rheumatoid arthritis. She told me that none of her toes on either foot had moved for fifteen years.

When the fifth routine was completed on her feet, she flexed all of her toes. She said, "A toe may seem like a very insignificant part of your body, but after fifteen years that sure feels good."

ADRENAL GLAND

There is one adrenal gland at the top of each kidney. This gland consists of two parts, one enclosing the other. The inner is called the medulla and it secretes adrenalin. The outer is called the cortex.

People have told me that their doctors said that the non-functioning of the adrenal was responsible for allergies. Some doctors have also said a faulty adrenal gland is the origin of anemia. When the sex glands cease because of the encumbrance of years, the adrenal assisted by the pituitary, should give the body such hormones as are needed to prevent it from immediately deteriorating into old age. If we find an elderly person looking much younger than they are it is invariably because of a strong pituitary and adrenal.

A woman in her late forties was suffering from an injured knee. She had been told that the cartilage over the end of the bone had been ruptured. It could be operated on, but then the joint would be stiff. She was having cortisone shots, and taking pain pills and sleeping medicine, and growing more desperate by the minute because she did not want the operation. A friend persuaded her to try the foot massages.

After twenty routines on her feet, she told me she was having no cortisone and no pain pills of any kind. When she was quiet, it no longer bothered her. She could stand and walk for a surprising length of time without discomfort.

I was startled when I looked at the feet of a man whose family had called me because he had asthma. All over his left foot and ankle he had sores which appeared similar to blisters.

I did not want to be offensive, but neither did I want to risk the danger of contagion. "Are you positive this is not a venereal infection?" I asked.

He told me that was exactly what the doctors had said when they first looked at his left foot, but all tests proved his body to be absolutely free from such a problem. One doctor believed that this was an allergy, although no other part of his body was similarly affected.

If today I were called on to massage such a foot I would do the work on the corresponding hand, but at that time I thought of nothing but the foot for the massage if it were there. I worked as best I could around the sores. I do not remember how many routines he had when he told me that all the sores had vanished and only the scars were left. He has since reported they never returned.

This same man was also suffering from enlarged testicles. His wife said they were so inflamed they would fill your doubled hands. The discomfort from them was so great he could scarcely sit or stand. The doctors had told her that because of his asthma and emphysema they did not see how he could live longer than three or four weeks and thought he could die any minute. More about his case history will be given in Chapter Ten.

One day as I was massaging the foot of this man up the kidney line with the adrenal at the top as given in Figures 4 and 5, he suddenly started writhing with intense agony. Naturally I stopped and wanted to know what had happened. A heavy sweat had broken out on his entire face.

He said he felt as if two huge hands had grabbed those sore testicles and wrung them. The same thing happened again when the next routine was given on his feet. Later he told me that from that minute those infected glands began to shrink and feel better. The improvement continued until they entirely ceased to bother him.

Another man, who was more than seventy years of age, was suffering from one infected testicle and from diabetes. He was in bed the greater part of the time, and his wife helped him to and from the bathroom.

He was given something like twenty-five massages on his feet. His wife told me he was never able to stop the insulin shots, but the testicle entirely quit bothering him. The last reports from him said that he was raking the yard and doing many other chores which are normal for a man of his age. He said he was enjoying life generally.

Three women who never knew each other were having similar problems. All were having hemorrhages during the menopause and had been told that a hysterectomy was the only answer. All had decided to try the foot massages. One found her feet cleared of the crystalline deposits at fourteen routines, one at sixteen, and one at twenty-five. Two reported that all bleeding had stopped and they were feeling fine. Later those two told me they were entirely through the menopause. The third said she had quit menstruating, but had gone to her doctor to make preparation for the hysterectomy. He examined her and told her she did not need an operation.

She reminded him, "You told me I needed an operation."

He answered, "When I told you that, you needed an operation. But you don't now."

So many young girls as well as women have told me that after the foot massages they experienced complete relief from discomfort at the time of their periods that I could not give the number without going back through my books to count them. One young woman had me massage her feet because of painful menstruation. After the first routine on her feet, she began to flow heavily and did not want me to touch her again. This continued for eleven days, then she called me and said, "Come and undo what you have started."

I went and gave her a complete massage on both feet, and immediately afterward she stopped. She decided we might as well continue and see what would happen. The third month from the time I first started on her feet, she called to tell me she was having a very normal flow with no pain.

A woman in her forties and a young woman of twenty both told me the same thing after their feet were cleared of crystals. Whereas in the past they had suffered horrible cramps with a scanty and irregular flow, they now had to watch the calendar and be prepared. If they were not, menstruation would start when they were totally unprepared.

Two women, who did not know each other, told me they had suffered from a fallen uterus. One said that hers would even drop down outside the vagina. One was quite skeptical about the foot massages. She said that in the past, when this problem bothered her, she had gone to a chiropractor. She said he would adjust her neck and back and she could feel that uterus draw up into position. Someone had told her that foot massages do the same, so she decided to try and find out if they would.

When I went to give her the sixth routine on her feet she said, "I just could not believe my own senses. I could actually feel that uterus moving back up where it belonged."

The other woman told me it seemed too good to be true, but her uterus had gone back into its proper position. The doctor of a young married woman had told her that she had a cyst on one ovary the size of a big orange. He assured her that she must have an operation, because a cyst of that size would never go away. She asked him to give her a month.

She called me. "Get down here and get busy on my feet. I don't want that operation."

She was the mother of the baby who could not sit up when it was ten months of age. Having seen what the massage had done for her son, had given her hope. Twice a week for that month she had the entire routine on her feet, and then she went back to her doctor for an examination before he would operate.

She said he told her, "I don't know what has happened to your cyst, but it's gone. It must have ruptured and come out with your menstruation, because if they break they will always bleed."

A mother was being given the foot massages when her daughter, who had ben married three or four months, asked me to massage her feet over the areas for female organs. It only required a few minutes to massage the spots (designated in Figure 6 and Figure 7 as the uterus and ovary).

The next time I saw these people they told me that about three hours after I left their house, a pain struck this young woman in the region of one ovary and she started bleeding from the vagina. All they could think of that might be wrong was a miscarriage, and they rushed her to the doctor.

He examined her, and told them that she was certainly fortunate because a big cyst, which had been on one of her ovaries, had ruptured and was draining. He told them that if this had not happened when it did, in the near future it would have been necessary to have removed it by an operation.

When one party was having her fourth foot massage, she told me she had been terribly frightened the next day after

106

the third routine on her feet. All at once she had started bleeding from the vagina, and something the size of her fist dropped out of her. She described it as a dark purplish mass. She was certain it could not have been a miscarriage because she had just ended her period.

I asked her what she did with it because I wanted her to show it to a doctor. She had been so excited she had flushed it down the drain. She said that two or three years previously the doctors had done a D and C on her and had told her that she had a fibroid tumor. They said at that time that when it became necessary to remove it they would do a complete hysterectomy. I wanted her to go back to the doctors and get their diagnosis of her situation now. She said, "Nothing doing. I'm not going through another dilation."

Another lady in her seventies had a similar experience. I had told her about the first woman, and she decided that if anything like that should happen to her she would be calm. She was sure she would save the object and take it to a doctor. However, when it happened, she did exactly like the first party. She said that when she saw the bleeding she became so excited she forgot everything else.

The mother of the baby which could not sit up at ten months of age was trying to give birth to another baby. For three weeks she had been having labor pains which would reach three minutes apart and then stop. Her doctor had put her in a hospital and given her medicine. He told her the birth was restrained by an infection in her body. However, there was no change and she was sent home to wait.

She called me. "I've worn out my husband and my dad and his wife because I can't sleep. They keep thinking any minute I'll go into hard labor, but I don't. Please come down here and do something for me."

She was given the complete routine on her feet. The next day they told me that her pains stopped as usual, but she began a heavy yellow discharge and then went to sleep. She slumbered so deeply she did not even hear her youngest child crying in the same room. The next morning she awakened feeling quite refreshed, there were no pains and the baby was not yet born.

Another complete routine was done on her feet. They told me that within an hour after I left, her pains started three minutes apart and became rapidly harder. She went to the hospital, and gave birth to the baby.

Another young woman urged me to give her the foot massages early in her pregnancy, but I refused because she had not previously experienced them. I feared that the sudden relaxation of her nerves might react unpleasantly on the pregnancy. If she had been given the manipulations before conception, then her entire body would have been accustomed to the reactions following the release of her nerves.

When the time came for her to be delivered, but the pains had not started, I gave in to her pleading and massaged her feet. Afterward she told everyone that was by far the easiest birth and the quickest, and she was determined that if she had another baby she was going to have a foot massage just before her pains started.

LYMPH GLANDS

The lymph which transudes from the capillaries resembles diluted blood plasma. It has a much greater responsibility in conveying the food to the tissues of the body for their consumption than does the blood. The lymph goes outside its vessels and literally bathes the cells with food.

The lacteals, the lymphatic, and the thoracic ducts are the vessels which convey the lymph through the body. Interposed in the path of the lymphatics are lymph glands through which the lymph filters much as coffee in a percolator. The purpose of these glands is to free the lymph from bacteria and other noxious materials. If too much is imposed on the lymph glands, then they themselves become infected and we have a situation known as mononucleosis.

The lymph has come from the blood and must return to it, or the tissues become water-logged with this otherwise very important fluid. This invokes a condition known as edema. The thoracic duct carries the lymph which it drains from the left side of the body to the junction of the left subclavian vein and the left jugular vein, where it is poured back into the blood. The right lymphatic duct carries the lymph which it drains from the right side of the body to the circulatory system at the union of the right subclavian vein and the right jugular vein.

The first professional massage I gave was on the feet of a young woman who had enlargd lymph glands on each side of her neck. They had been swollen for eight years, during which time she had received much medication with no change in the situation with the enlarged glands. She said that her family physician had told her he did not know how she lived, because there was not a gland in her body functioning as it should.

The night after she had been given this routine on her feet she said she had fever and felt as if red hot coals of fire were passing down the sides of her neck across her armpits and down the sides of her body. The next morning this was all gone. When she went into the bathroom to wash her face and looked into the mirror, she stood there gazing at herself with amazment. She could hardly believe her own eyes, because after all these years, she had lost hope that anything would ever take away those unsightly lumps from her neck. It was too good to be true, but every vestige of swelling had disappeared. Quite recently she told me it has not returned, and that was eight years ago.

A woman called me to give her fifteen-year-old daughter the foot massages. The doctor had told them that the enlargements on the girl's neck were infected lymph glands; but in one place, an inch wide, up and down the right side of her neck, was a tumor. He told them it must be removed by surgery.

They told me they were in no hurry to rush her into an operating room. If everything else failed, they would then think about it. They wanted her to have the foot massages and see what happened. When I went to give her the fifth routine, her mother met me at the door with the news that all the swollen lymph glands were completely reduced and the tumor was only half the size it had been.

After fourteen massages on her feet, she felt nothing but my thumb and fingers. Shortly afterward, the mother reported to me their joy that the tumor had completely disappeared. Three years later, they told me it had not returned.

A daughter had told me that her mother, who was an elderly woman in her eighties, had grown quite fat. When the first massage was begun on her feet, my thumb and fingers dented her foot as they might bread dough. Having read and studied as much as I had about the body I realized the indication, but not being a medical physician I could not diagnose. I inquired if her mother had seen a doctor recently. Since the elderly lady had not complained, they had not taken her to be examined. She had called me because her mother did not sleep well, and some friends told her they certainly could rest at night after the foot massages.

The next morning, after the first routine on the mother's feet, the daughter called me and said, "Now I know why you asked me if mother had seen a doctor. She was not fat. It was bloat. It had to be, but the massages are taking it down. This morning she is the most peculiar sight I have ever seen. Her face, neck, and arms are skinny, but the rest of her is as fat as a butterball."

The daughter wanted to know if the rest of the bloat would leave her mother. Of course all I could promise her was that time would tell. The daughter assured me later that the next morning, after each routine on her feet, the swelling would be further down her body, and then her legs, and last of all her feet. Then it was gone.

"Sleep," the daughter said, "Mother is sleeping like a

baby, and taking naps in the day and waking so refreshed."

I have given this about the lymph because the edema is caused by the lymph not returning to the blood as it should. However, it could quite properly be included in the heart and the circulatory system because, as I have been informed, it is the proper circulation of the blood which induces the natural return of the lymph.

LIVER AND GALLBLADDER

The liver is the largest gland in the body and is both exocrine and endocrine. An exocrine gland delivers, by way of a duct, its secretion to the part of the body where it is used. The endocrine emits into the bloodstreams the hormone which it creates. These hormones have a powerful effect on the body, such as controlling growth, shapes of the various members, and adjustment to outside influences.

From materials extracted from the blood, the liver cells form the bile. The secretion is drained from the liver through a tube which is joined by the cystic duct from the gallbladder to form a common bile duct which conveys this very important digestive fluid to the duodenum. There it performs a major work in the final preparation of the food for the use of the body. I have also been told it assists in the elimination of the feces from the colon.

The liver extracts harmful substances from the blood, either changing them into harmless or excreting them into the bile. In the later case, they are carried to the duodenum. It shoves them into the jejunum and they can pass into the ileum. There they may be picked up by the lymph, and be passed through the lymph glands where they should find a proper disposal, as has already been explained under "lymph."

If these harmful substances are absorbed into the blood through the walls of the small intestine, they then can still be destroyed by the white blood cells. If these obnoxious substances escape the liver, the lymph glands and the blood, there is still another avenue by which they may be kept from harming the body. If elimination is good, they can pass into the colon and be evacuated from the entire system. What a wonderful four-way plan for the human body, so that it may cope with all the detrimental substances which invade its privacy.

Again, our attention is drawn to the importance of the alimentary canal and all of the glands which give their assistance to its performances. Again, how important is the selection of that which enters our mouths as well as the manner in which it is taken. No small wonder that the human race is beset with cancer of the liver and the pancreas.

The liver also secretes fibrogen and antifibrogen, two hormones which are poured directly into the blood stream. The fibrogen causes the blood to clot easily outside the bloodstream, and the antifibrogen keeps it from clotting inside the blood stream. The purpose of each is apparent.

The author was born into a family that suffered much from the effects of sluggish liver glands. I myself, had typhoid fever at the age of six months and suffered from malarial chills as long as I lived in the mosquito-infested lowlands along the river. My husband ate the same food, drank the same water, and was bitten by the same mosquitoes, but did not know the feeling of a malarial ache.

Our old family doctor told me that the difference between my husband and me was a faulty and a normal liver. My legs were disfigured at a young age with unsightly lumps of bloodclots as well as varicose veins.

A friend told me that looking at the change in the clots and veins showing on my legs would lead her to believe that the body could receive much help from the foot massages. She said the most convincing one to her was a clot which was as big around as the ball of her thumb, and became a mere streak since I had been given the manipulations on my feet.

They also tell us that the liver has a great power of replacing cells which have been thrown out of action by disease. That is easy for me to believe, because a woman whom I know to be very truthful, and a person who is not guilty of exaggeration, told me the story of a man she knew.

He had been examined, and a test proved his liver to be malignant. He was told that the gland was too far gone to be repaired, and that he might as well be prepared to leave this life very shortly. He suddenly made the decision that he did not want to die at that time, and was going to do his best to make their prediction false. He quit drinking all alcoholic beverages, and stopped the use of tobacco in any form. He went to someone competent to advise him about nutrition, and immediately began to follow instructions.

The woman who told me about him said that at that time he had lived fifteen years after he was told that at the very best he only had a few months. Furthermore, he looked quite healthy and said he felt fine.

The people who complain of a faulty liver invariably tell me, after the first foot massages, that they will have spells of feeling so utterly weary that they do not even want to put one foot in front of the other. But when the crystalline deposits are gone from the feet, they report much more vigor and endurance.

The gallbladder is similar to a small storage tank for the bile and acts like a thermostat in portioning the secretion out into the cystic duct. A woman who called me had been told by her doctor that her gallbladder would eventually need to be removed because it had ceased to function. She decided she would try the foot massages first.

After about the third routine on her feet, she began to have terrible spells of nausea. She read in a book written by an herbalist about the value of using goldenseal and peppermint teas to relieve such conditions. Immediately she began to drink both, and continued with the foot manipulations.

After fourteen full routines had been done on her feet, she asked her doctor to give her a complete physical report.

She was admitted to a hospital, and three doctors thoroughly examined her, using all the tests and X-rays necessary to accomplish a complete diagnosis of her condition. One of the physicians was the man who had told her that the gallbladder must be removed. All three medical men agreed that her gallbladder was functioning perfectly.

If you are massaging a foot and the gallbladder area is quite sharp, inquire if the person has gallstones. If they have, stop the complete routine at once and do only the parathyroid, which will be caught in the areas marked thyroid in Figure 4 and Figure 5. Continue this for at least three weeks. If the person is not aware of any gallstones, caution them to let you know at once if they develop a sharp or unusual pain in the region of the liver or gallbladder.

I had once given a woman two foot massages when she had an attack of what she supposed was indigestion. To me, it sounded suspiciously like a gallbladder attack. I told her I was afraid that her nerves might be trying to dispose of something which should not be in the body.

"Go ahead and give me another routine. Rubbing my feet couldn't possibly cause that." She was firm, and I, being new in the work, was easily convinced.

I did not like what had just happened; but I had been told you could not hurt anyone with these massages, so I gave her another. The next day after that one, she had an attack which put her in the hospital. An X-ray showed her gallbladder to be full of stones. They wanted to operate, but she refused. They gave her medicine to stop the stones from trying to pass, and dismissed her.

She wanted me to give her another routine; but by this time I was thoroughly convinced that she should not have another one, and I was firm. For four weeks I massaged only the parathyroid areas, after which we continued the regular routines. Quite awhile afterward she told me she had no more trouble with her gallbladder.

PANCREAS

The pancreas is another gland which is both endocrine and exocrine. It secretes the pancreatic juice which goes through a passage to the common bile duct, and from there to the duodenum where it assists with the final digestion of food. It also is responsible for a hormone which goes directly into the bloodstream.

After the first one or two foot massages, diabetics invariably report to me that there is a decided increase of sugar showing in the urine; but when that causes them to go for a blood test, they are told that much less sugar is denoted in the blood.

A man who was taking insulin in an oral form called me to massage his feet. After about six or seven full routines he began to have dizzy spells. He went to his doctor and was given a blood test after which the doctor assured him that he was overassisted, and the physician told him to stop his medicine. He did, and the dizziness ceased. With no further problems, the massages were continued until he felt no discomfort when I massaged his feet.

I was called to the home of a woman who had psoriasis, and I found a most pitiful sight. She was lying on a sheet that was so clean it was snowy-white except for splotches of fresh blood scattered all over it. She was covered with an immaculate spread except for a few red stains on it.

She showed me her arms and legs. They as well as her hands, feet, and, entire body were totally covered with a solid mass of huge red bumps surmounted with thick layers of scales. Only her face was free from the psoriasis. Even the hair on her head was thick with it. The scales were so hard that the movements she made cracked them down into the flesh and from such places the blood was oozing. She told me she was bleeding from the rectum which also contained bumps and scales.

She had been afflicted in this fashion since she was fourteen, and she was now in her middle forties. It would leave her during the summer, and return some time in September. By Christmas she was always in such a condition that no attempt was made to dress her in even the flimsiest garment.

They would simply grease her all over the body with medicine the doctor prescribed and cover her with a sheet.

The doctors gave her no solution for her problem, she said, except to relieve the burning and itching with a medicine which resembled a salve. They told her it was caused by the pancreas which did not function properly. They were certain her nerves were causing that. She had heard that foot massages relieved and therefore normalized the nerves, so she was anxious to try them.

There was no way I could do the work except to massage over the scales. After the first routine she told me she was terribly nauseated, but the bleeding from the rectum had stopped.

After the fourth manipulation she told me she had a very frightening experience. The next morning she had awakened to discover her entire forehead had raised up in a huge lump of psoriasis, and there had never been any on her forehead.

The second morning after the fourth routine, she aroused with the sensation that there was nothing of her except her head and neck. She said she felt if her body was there it must be completely numb. It frightened her so that she gave a big flop like a fish and her body began to tingle all over.

She got up and went to the bathroom. She looked into the mirror, and stood there completely amazed. The lump of psoriasis which had come on her forehead the previous day was gone. She said from that day all bleeding stopped. The scales began to crumble and fall off. The lumps subsided in the center, first leaving the appearance of huge ringworms all over her.

The day I gave her the sixteenth routine she felt no sharpness whatever in her feet, and she told me there was not a particle of psoriasis anywhere on her body. Later she reported to me that she had the happiest Christmas of her life. For the first time in more than thirty years she was out of bed on Christmas Day. She not only cooked dinner for her family, but also had guests which she was so thrilled to be able to invite. She said it was wonderful to live like a normal human again.

KIDNEYS

In previous chapters I have stressed the fact that these compression massages should not be given more frequently than twice a week. I would like to make two exceptions. The story I will tell here, and one in Chapter Eleven, will explain the reason.

In Chapter Two, I told you about a woman with diabetis who had had half of each foot amputated and I massaged her hands. After three or four routines, she had a kidney infection and was forced to go to the county hospital. When they dismissed her, and she was back home, I went to see how she was feeling.

She said she was in so much pain she did not know what to do with herself. Her kidneys had not voided more than a few drops for forty-eight hours. She had been dismissed by doctors, and she wanted me to do the complete massage on her hands. I decided to do only the areas designated on the charts as kidney, ureter tube, and bladder.

The next day she told me that all night the urine passed from her in large quantities, but had almost stopped again. The manipulations were again given on the kidney, ureter tube and bladder lines. The next day she reported that the kidneys flushed freely again. After a week of daily massage on the kidney, ureter tube, and bladder areas, she told me her problem of voiding had entirely ceased. The regular routine twice a week was then continued.

The experience occurred early in my work as a foot masseuse, and from that time, anyone who called me and was having a similar problem, was given work on the kidney, ureter tube, and bladder areas only every day for a week. If it was a man, the prostate area was included because the prostate gland is wrapped around the urethra. At the present time there has been only one person who has not reported complete relief after this procedure.

If a kidney line on the foot has extremely sharp crystals, I always ask the recipients if they have kidney stones. If they do not know, I ask them to watch the urine for any change in it, and if they find anything different to report to me immediately. A case early in this work caused me to take that precaution.

I had given a man, who lived alone, these foot massages. When I went to do the fourth routine on his feet, he was not there. I was surprised, because he was always punctual. He was a businessman who often went out of town, so I thought that perhaps he had been unexpectedly called away and could not reach me by phone.

Since there was nothing I could do until he contacted me, I went on to my other customers. Two or three days later, when I came in from work, my husband told me that someone had called for me from a hospital and had left the telephone number. It was this man.

He said that after the first foot masage he had begun to pass gravel in the urine, but had never once thought there might be a possibility that the manipulations on his feet were causing it so he had not mentioned this fact to me. The climax came when a stone, which was so large it could hardly pass, began to move down the ureter tube. He said he felt as if he would die before the stone passed from him.

He said, "It was terrible, but I'm glad it is out."

From that time, if the crystals are extremely sharp in those areas, I question the party carefully. If I feel there is the least danger of a repetition of this man's experience, I stop everything on the feet immediately except the parathyroid.

Since others have not felt that they have discovered a definite portion for the parathyroid, I massage the entire thyroid as shown in Figures 4 and 5.

I have already told about the polio victim who said that after the foot massages something which resembled ice crystals passed from her. The elderly lady whose daughter thought she was overweight when she had edema reported something passed in her urine which was very similar to flakes from the inside of an orange peeling.

She said that for a day or two afterward her sides were very sore in the part of the body where the ureter tubes extend from the kidneys to the bladder. Within three or four days that tenderness subsided. Nothing more of that nature happened with her although she had something like eighteen full routines on her feet.

Chapter Ten

BRONCHIAL TUBES AND LUNGS

The abuse of the alimentary canal was stressed in Chapter Six, but may it be said here that it is probably no more neglected and abused than the bronchial tubes and lungs. Much is written and spoken on the subject of "smog." Perhaps very little can be done by the average individual except, at every opportunity, to take himself as far away from it as possible.

Quite a bit can be done by everyone to strengthen the respiratory system. This past week my eighteen-year-old grandson, who had come to visit me for two days, told me that shortly after arriving he had a slight chest cold. I gave him a complete foot massage, and the next morning I asked him how his lungs felt. He assured me they were fine.

Since he and his brother were going fishing, and the air was damp and cool, I wanted complete assurance about his chest and asked him to stand up and breathe to the bottom of his lungs. He stood up and began a deep inspiration, but stopped shortly. He contended there was no pain or actual discomfort. He was not accustomed to breathing so deeply and it was not easy.

He does not use tobacco, liquor, or dope. He is in college, and works outside of school hours; but that incident told me that he was not having all the exercise he needed. So much is written and spoken on activity of the body to reduce, beautify, and develop the appearance of the physique, but I would like to stress the same for the health of the individual. I will give you here a little exercise for the chest, which I have found quite strengthening to the lungs.

Locate a place where the air is as fresh as possible. Stand erect, hands hanging at the sides. I call this the chest lift, and that is exactly what we intend to accomplish. The idea is to fill the lungs to their greatest capacity of intake in three lifts, or we might call them hitches. The first part of the inspiration lifts the chest one-third of the way. The second brings it up two-thirds, and the last lifts the chest as high as it can go and fills the lungs and corresponding tubes with every particle of air they can possibly contain. Exhale slowly.

If before you have come near to the third part of this exercise you feel dizziness, stop at once. Later do the first part, and repeat each day until you feel you can safely add the second rise of the chest. When you can comfortably do one and two of this, then try all three. If you feel giddiness or any other warning symptom, it is not a sign you should not have this exertion but rather a signal of a desperate need for it. However, do remember that a starving body can be killed with too much food at first. In this fashion, too much exercise thrown on any part of the physique suddenly can bring disaster.

At seventy-one, I find this chest lift not only stimulating but also pleasant. I have been using it for quite a few years. It might interest you to know that in a physical test which was being given to me by a medical doctor, during which time he was listening to my lungs and telling me to breathe thus and so, he made a comment on the strength of my respiratory organs.

He said, "A tuberculous growth would certainly have a hard life in your lungs." He told me that my chest was really strong.

To make discussion of the lungs easier, see Figure 29.

When breathing is mentioned, we often think of only the intake of oxygen and the expelling of carbon dioxide. But try this little experiment.

Sit in quiet silence, breathing in slow, regular rhythm for

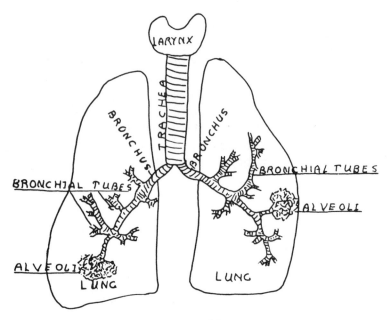

Fig. 29

three or four minutes. Now feel your pulse. For the next few
seconds breathe staccato. Notice how your pulse becomes
rapid and irregular. I once read an article written by a doctor, who said he was convinced that good breathing habits
not only regulated the heartbeats but also strengthened the
organ itself.

BRONCHITIS

Bronchitis is a condition in which there is an inflammation
of the bronchi or bronchioles. A little girl who was about a
year and a half old had suffered all of her existence with this
problem. On two occasions she had almost lost her life before getting relief.

She was having another attack and the mother and the
grandmother had just gone through three harrowing days

and nights with her. She was being given the medicine which they always used, but she could not sleep and did not play. Since this had repeated itself so often, they were desperate.

They knew quite a few people who had been given the foot massages, and they had heard the reports given afterward. It made them wonder if it might help in her case and they told me they wanted to try them for their young child.

It was difficult to decide if the baby was crying from the discomfort of the crystals cracking or from pure fright. By the time I had completed the manipulations on the right foot and was well started on the left one, the little girl was sound asleep. She would flinch nervously as my thumb went over various spots, but she did not waken.

Later, they told me she slept for two hours after I was gone. She got up and played with her toys for an hour and a half, and then went back to bed and slumbered soundly all night.

The next time I went to massage her feet, they told me what happened the next morning after she had that good night of rest. Quite unexpectedly and suddenly her fever shot up, and she started coughing and choking. They ran with her to a pay telephone. The grandmother called the doctor, while the mother was holding the child.

The mother told me that huge chunks of phlegm started coming from the child's mouth. The mother, being otherwise unprepared, caught the stringy mucus until it filled her doubled hands. As suddenly as it had begun, the ordeal ended. The little girl was calm and there was no indication of fever or other distress. Since the grandmother had already contacted the doctor, and he had told her to bring the little one in, they went on to his office.

He made an examination and assured them that her lungs were perfectly clear. He said she might have a little in her sinuses, but otherwise she was in fine condition. She was given about six routines on her feet. That was six years ago, and recently the grandmother told me that the child never suffered another attack.

A boy of eight seemed to always be sick with an infection in his bronchial tubes. He had a little hacking cough which his family believed was a habit. He had been scolded, bribed, and punished, but the cough persisted. He had a poor appetite, and was thin and pale.

They called for me to come and massage his feet. After the third routine the coughing stopped, and the last report they gave me, it had not returned. His appetite had increased as well as his weight. They said there was nothing spectacular, but just a general improvement. At one time he was caught in a hard downpour of rain and they fully expected to need the doctor and maybe even the hospital. To their complete surprise, no problem followed. They said that something had happened to change him completely, or that exposure would have brought him near to death.

BRONCHIECTASIS

Bronchiectasis is an enlargement of either or both bronchi. It may be a sequel to a disease such as bronchitis, tuberculosis, or pneumonia. I have been told by some of its victims that it is treated by getting an antiseptic into the affected passages either by inhalation or injection.

A seventeen-year-old girl had suffered all her life with bronchiectasis. Her parents had come to the end of their mental faculties. Should they take her here, or would it be best to go there? She had been everywhere, to all the best clinics, and still she could do none of the things other girls enjoyed. Worse than that, it seemed that her very life was threatened every day.

The doctors had warned her she must never go into the bathroom, turn on the hot water, and close the door. The steam might cause suffocation before she could get out. Her older married sister lived in California, but she could never visit her because she could not risk her life in so much humidity. She could not be present at many entertainments because of the flower decorations. The girl told me she had such a fuzzy feeling in her brain most of the time that she could not think well and it made school most difficult.

In desperation they decided they might as well try the foot massages. Nine routines on her feet were done, and she felt nothing but my thumb and fingers. She told me that the fuzzy feeling had left her brain and the heavy oppression, as if a weight rested on her chest, was no longer there. She said she had gone into the bathroom and, without remembering the warning of the doctors, she had closed the door. When she recalled what they said she was frightened; but on second thought she realized she was not in the least suffocated, so she did not open the door.

She said it was as if a new life had opened before her. She visited her married sister in California and thoroughly enjoyed the association. All this was seven years ago. The mother says that the daughter is now married and living a completely normal life.

A woman in her seventies had been afflicted with bronchiectasis for a number of years. After the first massage, she told me she could not believe her own sense when she awakened the next morning to find the sun shining brightly and realized she had not awakened a single time that night with a necessity to cough.

She said it was wonderful to have a good night's rest again. Later she reported a decided improvement in her condition but did not claim a complete recovery, as did the seventeen-year-old girl.

ASTHMA

In asthma, the little bronchioles shrink which causes the alveoli or air cells to be too crowded together to contain a proper amount of air. Naturally that makes the breathing difficult, and in extreme or progressed cases impossible, resulting in death.

One day I received a telephone call pleading for me to come quickly to a certain house where I had never been. As usual, I had appointments throughout the day, but the party who had called told me I must come at once because I was so badly needed. As I knew the person who had called quite well, and had already done much work for his family, I made other arrangements with some of the people who had already engaged my services for that day.

The man for whom I had been called had been in the hospital three days but had been dismissed. He had medicine for his asthma, but it looked as if every breath might be his last. When I walked into the room, he was slumped in a sitting position with his head leaning over in his wife's lap. From utter exhaustion he was sleeping, but every breath was so labored it appeared as if it might be his last.

Four or five sympathetic neighbors were sitting in the room. It was no time for explanations about the type of massage I do. As I had driven to this house I had prayed for wisdom to handle any situation I might find when I arrived.

With the help of those around me, I got him into a sitting posture on the divan and we propped him up with pillows. I began the routine on his feet. When I reached the line marked "back" in Figure 4, he suddenly began the most peculiar behavior and I was afraid to even think of what might be happening to him.

His wife cried out, "He's breathing to the bottom of his lungs."

Then I realized that the sudden relief of filling his chest with air had been too much for his nerves, and he was in a state of hysteria. What could I do next? I had heard a sudden slap on the cheek would stop it; but, of course, I would not do that in this case.

I clapped my hands in front of his face and said, "Stop it."

That did the trick, and he came out of it weeping but soon regained his self-control. "Oh," he said, "That was the most wonderful thing in the world—to be able to breathe like that after what I've been through."

"She only rubbed your foot," one of the women remarked. "What in the world could that do?"

"All I know is I can breathe as I haven't done for days."

His wife spoke up. "I'd say you haven't breathed that easily for months."

Everyone in the room was relieved but puzzled and full of questions. It took a long time to finish the manipulations on his feet, and answer the inquiries. The thing that perplexed them most was that it was so simple. The man followed me to the door and could hardly allow me to leave for telling me over and over what a miracle had just been performed on him, and how ridiculous it would sound to those who had not seen it.

Another man's wife had been told by some very good doctors that he could not live more than three weeks because of asthma and emphysema. Furthermore, they thought it was possible that he might go any minute. She had called me to give her the foot massages; and while I was going over her feet, he was in the room struggling for every breath he drew. She said she had pleaded with him to try the foot massages, but he had refused. He knew it could not help him, and he was too sick to be bothered.

When I was through with her, she turned to him. "Why don't you try it just once?" He submitted as if it might be easier to submit than to argue with her.

As I went over his feet he gradually became quiet. The pastor of his church dropped in to see him shortly before I finished. From other members of his congregation the preacher had heard about these manipulations and asked him how he felt.

"I don't know anything about it except I was sure having a rough time trying to get air into my lungs when she started, but it's perfectly easy now. That's enough for me. I'm going to have some more of this."

It took quite a number of massages to clear the crystals from his feet, but he told me he never had any real problem with his asthma after that first day. Six years later, I heard from some of his family that he was having no more trouble with his lungs and had even sung in the church choir.

I hope you will notice that the reactions of the recipient in this next story are entirely different. This man's family had urged him for a year to try these massages because of his asthma and emphysema, but he not only flatly refused but ridiculed the entire idea.

Finally he became so weak he could not stand up long enough to wash his face and hands, and told his wife to call me. When I began to massage his feet I told him that if he felt the least difference of any kind within his body to tell me at once. I had completed the routine on his right foot, and on the left foot I was working along the area which is the shortest line marked "back" in Figure 6, when he told me he suddenly felt cold all over as if he had a chill.

I stopped at once, and in a second he was fighting for his breath in an asthma attack. I asked for his inhaler, and he pointed toward the refrigerator. I ran to it, found the inhaler, and he used it. It did not work as rapidly as we, who were watching, longed for it to do, but gradually it did ease him.

Now that he had started he was determined to see these massages through to end the crystals in his feet. Each time I could not complete the routine because he would repeat the chilling and difficulty in breaking. At last the day came when he was given the entire massage on both feet. Even then a little difficulty with his breathing began and he was forced to use the inhaler. Then the day came when the manipulations were accomplished on both feet without the aid of the inhaler. It required eighteen routines before he felt nothing but my thumb and fingers.

It was then he told me that he was using no inhaler and no medicine, and had no difficulty with his breathing. Shortly afterward his wife told me he was back at work. He is a vegetable inspector, and in the course of his labor walks across fields and climbs trucks.

Three months after that, he was given six more foot massages. Afterward he was checked regularly twice a year, and each time had six routines on his feet.

The day came when after six months he still felt no crystals in his feet, so I did not check him any more. I have not even seen the man for more than four years, but have talked with him by phone within the past few months. He assured me he was doing fine and working despite the fact that he was coming close to seventy years of age.

From the time I gave that man the first foot massage I have never started on the feet of anyone who has asthma and uses an inhaler without it lying beside us as I work. It would be my advice to anyone else doing this work to take the same precaution. This last man does not hesitate to tell others that these massages saved his life, and he also admits he had suffered some rough reactions before the victory was won.

He also says, "Nobody needs to be in a worse shape than I was. When you are so weak you can't stand long enough to wash your face and hands, you are in pretty bad shape."

EMPHYSEMA

In the case of emphysema, the walls of the little alveoli lose their elasticity. The person thus afflicted can draw a breath in, but is unable to force the air out. The walls gradually atrophy and go to pieces, leaving large sacks instead of the normal small cells. As all of us know, this can and often does result in death.

Both of the men whose stories I have just related were diagnosed as being in the advanced stages of emphysema. I never have and never will make any claims of having cured anything. I am simply repeating what they and their wives told me.

The first of these men said that he went back to the clinic after his feet were free from any feeling of cracking crystals. Three of the same doctors examined him again. They told him to stand up and breathe to the bottom of his lungs. He did that. They told him to exhale. That was accomplished without even a wheeze. He told me that the doctors said, "Something has happened to you that we certainly did not expect."

One woman told me she had emphysema brought on by pneumonia. I do not remember too much about the work with her, because there was nothing that seemed to be outstanding. The thing I do remember is that she called me to say that she was having no more trouble with emphysema.

A party called me because her husband had emphysema. She said she knew he was dying of cancer on his kidney. He had been examined at a veteran's hospital, and they had told her the malignancy was too far advanced to do anything about it. He had been sent home to take medicine for relief until he should reach a stage when he would be forced to return to the hospital for care.

The wife said she knew that the foot massages could do nothing for the cancer on his kidney, but someone had told her what this work had done for their emphysema.

She told me she knew he had to go, but she did not want to see him suffer the way she had heard they could at the end. Perhaps half a dozen routines were done on his feet. He vowed that not only the emphysema was better, but the pain in his back was also better. For a time he refused to take his pain medicine. Later she told me that he passed away but not from the emphysema, for which she was thankful.

CHAPTER ELEVEN

HEART AND CIRCULATORY SYSTEM

In Chapter Ten there is a paragraph on breathing habits, in which an article by a doctor was mentioned. In this doctor's opinion, good breathing exercises not only helped the lungs but also strengthend the heart. No organ in the body can be invigorated with any type of activity unless that portion is well nourished. So whatever we consider on the subject of the body we are always led back to the consideration of wholesome food.

A heart specialist in Phoenix told a friend of mine that heart attacks originated more from that which was put into the mouth of the individual than from exertion of the body.

In Ecclesiastes, the human heart is compared with a pitcher at a fountain or a wheel at a cistern. In our day it could be better understood if explained as working similar to the pump at a filter plant because it persistently drives the blood through the body.

The blood carries food from the digestive tract and oxygen from the lungs to the portions of the body where it can be utilized. It is responsible for the waste matter reaching the lungs, skin, and kidneys, where it can be expelled from the body. It acts very much like an internal transportation system for the hormones which control chemical activities.

This important fluid is composed of three-fifths plasma and two-fifths cells. The red blood cells number seven hundred to one white cell. The purpose of the red blood corpuscles is to carry oxygen. The white cells, being fewer in number, are larger. They protect the body from disease germs,

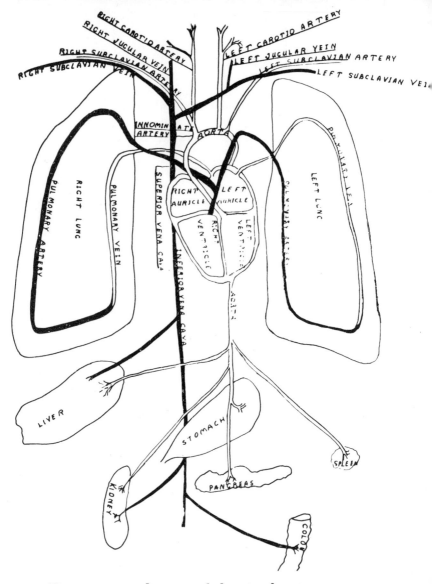

Figure 30 is a diagram of the circulatory system.
DIAGRAM OF HEART AND CIRCULATORY SYSTEM
= indicates pure blood in blood vessels ▬ indicates impure
blood

promote tissue repair, and aid in absorption of food from the intestines.

Our family physician gave me an example of the work of the white blood cells, which I would like to pass on to you. He took, for example, a boil. He said it began with the attack of a germ on some portion of the surface of the body. The inflammation and swelling were produced by the rush of the white blood cells, like good soldiers, to the scene of the action. When the fight was over and the victory won by the white corpuscles, the yellowish eruption which came forth was made up of white blood cells which lost their lives in the battle.

In the foot massage, two experiences reminded me of the description given by our doctor. After three routines had been done on a woman's feet, she began to complain of a pain in her jaw. I suggested that it might be from a tooth, but she was certain it could not be. "I don't even have a cavity," she bragged.

The pain persisted, and became worse with each massage. Finally she went to a dentist, and the jaw was X- rayed. There was a cavity and an abscess at the root of a tooth which had every appearance of being perfect above the gum.

After a few manipulations on his feet a man told me he had an enlarged place, resembling a tumor, which had arisen on one testicle. He described it as being very painful and tender. It surprised and puzzled me, because I had never had a report of anything like that after the foot massages. After the next routine on his feet it was worse and after the third he was suffering so much pain that he went to see a specialist.

The swollen place was not a tumor and it was not on a testicle. It was an enlargement of the prostate. The doctor told him that the gland had been infected without his knowledge for quite some time.

The massages were stopped for two weeks while he was

taking medicine to kill the infection. When he was released by the specialist, the routines were continued on his feet. He was enthusiastic and grateful for this work.

According to our doctor's description of the work of the white blood cells, it must have been the rush of them which had caused the swelling. This man said that if these foot massages had not stirred his body to better action he might have gone on unaware of the infection until it had reached an unmanageable stage.

Fever may be produced by poisonous substances in the blood, invasion of germs, faulty metabolism, injury to tissues, constipation, uremia, or hysteria. One party told me that her doctor said that asthma was much harder to handle if it was not accompanied by fever. He explained his statement by telling her that if there was no fever it was a very good sign that the body had no fighting capacity.

Artery means air bearer, and was thus named because the first ones discovered were in a dead body and had nothing but air in them. All arteries go from the heart, as you will see in Figure 30, but they do not all carry pure blood. All veins go to the heart, but not all carry impure blood, as you may also notice in Figure 30.

If you have read in Chapter Nine about the hormones produced by the pituitary gland, you know that the walls of the blood vessels are kept healthy by this secretion. If the pituitary is not performing its normal function, the blood vessels may shrink. In this case the blood presure is forced to rise in order to pump the blood through the shrunken vessels, causing what is known as high blood pressure. On the contrary, if the pituitary is not functioning correctly, the walls of the arteries may stretch and cause low blood pressure.

High blood pressure can bring on arteriosclerosis, or hardening of the arteries in which cholesterol forms along the inside walls of the vessel. When I was studying this foot massage, my husband was quite skeptical. He asked me, "Don't you think there is a lot of imagination about this?"

I did not answer, because he was making a statement of his feelings rather than an inquiry. A few nights later, when he was preparing for bed and had removed his shoes, I walked over, took hold of his foot and cracked a crystal or two with the turn of my thumb.

He complained rather loudly about the pain, but I told him that if he was to really know anything about this he must allow me to try it on him. He consented. I was at that time very unlearned on the subject, but as best I could I went over his feet. When I stopped, he said his toes tingled as if they had been asleep and were just awakening.

For a number of years he had complained of a numbness in his feet. He had asked different doctors about it, and they all gave him the same answer: they assured him that this condition accompanied hardening of the arteries.

Two days after I had massaged his feet he became quite excited. He said all the numbnes had left his feet. Knowing his former skepticism I sat and smiled at him in a way that seemed to irritate him.

"And its not imagination either," he told me emphatically.

CORONARY THROMBOSIS

You will notice that in Figure 30, the blood vessels arise from the heart in an arched position. Coronary means pertaining to or resembling a crown, hence anything occurring in this area of the blood vessels is known as coronary. A thrombosis is the formation of a clot in the bloodstream, causing a local stoppage of the circulation. Reports from doctors and clinics give the coronary thrombosis as a leading heart problem.

A man called me to inquire about these foot massages. He wanted to know if they would do anything for impotency. He was in his early fifties, and did not think he should be troubled with such a problem at his age. I told him I had heard a doctor say that if there was no physical problem, impotency came from nerve bankruptcy. Of course I gave him the answer I always give. This was a massage, and it relieved tension of the nerves. I was new in this work or I would have inquired about the health of his entire body.

What I did not know was that this man had been in the hospital for three months because of coronary thrombosis and had not been able to go back to his occupation since. Without telling me about his heart problem, he decided he would have the manipulations on his feet.

The first time he went back for a check with his doctor after the routines on his feet were begun, he told me that the doctor cut down on his medicine. It was then I was informed of his coronary.

The man's doctor kept cutting down on his heart medicine. After he had been given fifteen complete routines on his feet, he went for another examination of the condition of his circulatory system. This time his medicine was stopped completely and he was told he could go back to his manual labor. After the sixteenth massage, when he felt nothing but my thumb and fingers going over his feet, he told me his normal sexual powers had been completely restored.

Another man had been told by his doctor that one of his heart valves was almost incapable of its normal action. He was cautioned and told he must quit work at once. He was also given medicine. He told his wife to call me. He was in such a weakened condition that I was fearful of doing much work on his feet. I did only the pituitary and adrenal at first, and little by little added other areas until at last, after many days, a complete routine was accomplished.

Slowly he gained strength. After six or eight months, the same doctor who had told him that his heart valve was practically gone assured him that the same valve was functioning quite well. That was three years ago.

This man is in his sixties, and he is careful not to strain himself lifting, but otherwise he does lots of physical work and is able to enjoy life generally.

ANGINA ATTACKS

When I was called to see a lady I will refer to as A. F., I took one look and feared to touch her. She was lying on her bed where, I was told, she remained the greater part of the time. Her face was without any normal color. Her voice was weak and often had a choking sound.

They told me she could not have company for an hour but she would suffer a heart attack afterward. Some time previously she had suffered a coronary and been in the hospital for quite a length of time. Since then she had experienced many anginas. She had low blood sugar, thyroid problems, a terrible condition of the colon, and her kidneys and bladder were often infected.

She had been told by a very close friend about a man who was near death and had been given these foot massages. He had grown steadily better and was now back at work. The friend had also told A. F. it was I who had done the manipulations on his feet. Because of all his, A. F. wanted desperately to have the routines done for her.

Having been told of the impoverishment of her body I hesitated because I was casting about in my mind for some benign way to bow out of the situation. The thought was foremost with me of the position I would be in if I should touch her and she should die under my hands. I began to suggest it was most unlikely that in her case anything would be accomplished with the foot massages.

I was sitting beside her bed, and she put out her weak hand and laid it upon my arm. Her plaintive voice, and the hopelessness of her dull eyes, pleaded along with her words. "Please try. You are my last hope. The doctors have told me they have done all they can. They tell me I do not respond to anything like anyone else. They don't say it, but I know they will be relieved when I'm gone and they don't have to hear from me again. Please don't turn me down."

I will never forget her eyes and her voice. Silently I asked

137

God to give me wisdom. I began with massage on the feet in the areas of the neck, back, pituitary, adrenal, kidney and bladder, as designated in Figure 4 and Figure 5. Previously, in Chapter One, reactions have been discussed slightly and further, in the case of asthma, in Chapter Nine. In coronary cases, no reactions which occurred had any unpleasant effects on the heart.

I had been told, by those who were in this work long before I began, that a digging massage, around the lower half of the seventh cervical or big bone at the base of the neck, had brought avowals of complete relief from a heart attack by the recipient. I had also been warned of disastrous results from the same massage around the upper half of the same vertebra. In boxing, a stroke from above down on the same bone is called a lethal blow and is illegal.

In Chapter Eight is the story of the woman with heart and nerve spells. After she had received the "digging" massage around the lower half of the seventh cervical, she declared it was as if she had been given oxygen.

In the case of A. F. she called me the next day, after she had been given the manipulations mentioned above. She was having an angina, and her medicine did not relieve it. The massage around the lower half of the cervical bone did nothing. Knowing that nerves to the heart also came from the area of the first, third, fourth and fifth thoracic vertebrae, I tried the digging manipulation on those bones with a motion which worked from below up.

When the fifth thoracic bone was reached, she assured me it gave her wonderful relief. After a few seconds of this massage with the digging upward motion, she told me the pain was entirely gone from her right arm and her chest.

For months and months this was repeated. I showed her that she had a sore spot in the line of the breastbone and level with the top of her breasts as well as in another tender place just beneath the lower end of the sternum. By massaging these two places with a circular motion she could sometimes relieve the pain in her chest and right arm to a certain extent until I could arrive to do the rubbing along the backbone.

For four months I was in the home of A. F. at least once but more often twice each day. For six or eight months her call for the massage on her backbone was expected any minute. All the people whose feet I massaged knew that if she called, I would quit on the second and go to her as fast as traffic lights and speed limits would permit.

Over and over I tried to teach her husband to do the massage along her backbone line but always she complained that he shut off her air instead of increasing it. At last the day came when she told me he was beginning to relieve her in that way. She said she was improving, and could be up the greater part of the day.

Then she announced that she had cooked dinner for company. She was again attending church, and doing her own grocery shopping. She even did her own washing and hung the clothes on the line. She said she had to be careful of too much reaching and lifting, but she could do a certain amount. These reports were given a year and a half or more after the first manipulations on her feet. During that time, the routines were given regularly twice a week.

Before I knew her, she had suffered from skin cancers on her face and neck. About the time it seemed she was going to be able to enjoy life again, the cancer problem on her face and neck flared up.

The foot massage was stopped while she was given treatment for the malignancy. That required a lengthy period of time, and her heart began to give her trouble again. Although she tried grapefruit juice, creosote tea, and red-clover-blossom tea, and dessert tea, from all of which other people had claimed the complete disappearance of cancers, hers hung on and presented quite a difficult matter.

At last she was dismissed by all the doctors who treated the cancers, and the foot massages were continued. The first of last June, I left Phoenix in order to find enough seclusion to write this book. She did rather well without the manipulations on her feet until sometime in August, when her heart began to distress her again.

About two weeks ago, just before Christmas, she called me and said that she must have me at once regardless of what I was doing. The partial massage was begun. I have just talked with her this morning and she assured me that she felt slightly better. It appears that she can never quit these manipulations so long as her life continues.

CEREBRAL HEMORRHAGE

At the present time these routines on the feet are being given to a lady in her eighties, and a man in his middle forties, both of whom have suffered strokes. The daughter-in-law of the lady told me that she was amazed when she saw her mother-in-law lift her paralyzed leg and cross it over the other leg after she had been given two of the complete routines on her feet. She said it was the first time that that leg had moved since the stroke six months previously.

The wife of the man told me that his left hand had hung in helpless inactivity since his stroke until six massages had been done on his feet. He had also discovered he could now snap the fingers of that hand quite well. She said she had noticed that he was often using the paralyzed hand without seeming to be conscious of doing this.

Chapter Twelve

CONSCIOUSLY RELAXING NERVOUS TENSION

So many people have asked me how, at my age, I can work for so many hours and continue to enjoy such good health that a public answer might be in order. May I stress that I am not giving any mental advice or making any recommendations. I am merely saying that there are some simple rules which I follow.

ARGUMENT

I have found that the most friendly argument can have a most jarring effect on my complete nervous system. Study the life of Jesus of Nazareth in the Bible, and you will find that He never argued. He counseled or taught, if He was given a receptive ear. If not, He remained calm and silent. They could coldly turn away from Him, or they could rave at a quiet individual who refused to be disturbed by their foolishness.

When someone wishes a word-battle with me, I have a rule which I follow. Either aloud or in the seclusion of my mind I say, "Have it your way."

If they continue to try to bestir me, I remain silent. The most persistent will eventually hush up if there is no response. It is perfectly easy not to speak and yet be mentally combative. I find that as devastating to my nrves as a word battle. To avoid it, I have developed a technique of hearing the words without allowing them to penetrate. I have been asked how I accomplish this.

If you can convince yourself you do not care what that

party thinks, you have it made. It is similar to a strange pup barking at your heels. You hear him, but you utterly disregard him. That causes the barking to lose its attraction for him.

One time, because I had studied the Bible extensively, I was invited to a so-called home Bible study along with two other guests of different faith. The others requested to come were men, and in no time at all they were shaking their fists at each other and using some very unbecoming words to describe their ideas of the stupidity of the opposing party.

If for no other reason, I would not have participated because of the damage it would have done to my nerves. I sat there and relaxed while they waged a war which in appearance resembled a TV comedy. When at long last it was over and they had departed, the hostess turned to me.

She said, "I'm disappointed. I invited you here because I had hoped you could lay them both in the shade, but you sat there like a stump."

I told her I was certain that my nerves were in far better condition than those of either of the men.

ONE WHO NAGS

As a child I grew up in a home where the wife nagged from the time she opened her eyes in the morning until she closed them at night. Otherwise my stepmother had some very admirable qualities, and I must give her credit for the fact that she eventually overcame this defect to a great extent.

From her I learned much about nervous control, because I either had to bend or break under her constant barrage of criticism. She had married my father when I was four years of age. Early in that experience with her, I determined that when I grew up I would cut out my tongue before I would be a nagger.

It has been my observation that critical people originate

from three types of personalities. Some are egotistical and self-centered; some have a terrific inferiority complex and must constantly wear others down in order to lift themselves up; and still others are perfectionists for the entire human race.

Whatever the category, the best antidote I have found for the sake of self-preservation is to put as many miles between myself and them as possible. Along these lines the *Proverbs of Solomon* give such adages as: "It is better to dwell in a corner of the housetop than in a wide house with a brawling woman." Also, "It is better to dwell in the wilderness than with a contentious and an angry woman."

Suppose you are trapped as I was. At least I was trapped until I was grown, so I was forced to soliloquize on the subject. I tried to understand and sympathize with my stepmother. If she was just egotistical, maybe I was a wee bit that way myself. In high school, I received my lesson in that.

My themes, as our writings were then called, easly held first place in the class and I was beginning to really admire myself. One day, a little slip of a girl moved in from Texas —and gave me a back seat in English class. At first I was chagrined, to say the least; and then I saw myself for what I really was—a very ordinary run-of-the-mill person.

Nothing better could have happened to me. In so many words, I could not better the other person, but I might learn lessons from even a nagger. So I learned to pity instead of despise.

LOSS OF A LOVED ONE

The loss of a loved one leaves a gap in our existence which in someway must be bridged, or, better yet, filled. Again I speak of my own experiences because I have given up parents, grandparents, uncles, aunts, a son, and a husband. Death is such a final thing which no amount of suffering on our part can change.

I can hear someone say, "But no one can take their place."

That is one hundred percent true. When I was forced to bow before the fate that had bereaved me, I began to think that perhaps if I had done this, or not done that, everything would have been different. I immediately closed my mind on that thought because it could do nothing but torture me.

Others whom I loved were trying to lift me up and help me to go on; for their sakes, I had to overcome my grief. I began by putting everything which had belonged to the departed one out of my sight. It was not disrespect for the dead. It was preservation of the living. Even pictures were stowed away. When I could see them without tears, I would bring them out again.

Above everything else, I kept away from the cemetery. After all, what comfort to them was to be found there? I much preferred to remember them as they had lived. I repeatedly told myself that there were many things much worse than death.

I realized I was really mourning for myself and not for them. I faced the fact that we cannot live with the dead. I determined to turn to the living and occupy my complete thoughts with them. I would be so usurped with the present that there would be no time left for the past.

RELAXED WALKING AND WORKING

We read much about jogging and walking in order to preserve muscle tone, but I have not read anything about relaxed walking to help the nerves. I try to make it a part of my daily program.

In doing this relaxed exercise, keep the mind as nearly vacant as possible. To accomplish this, do not notice anything about you. Move the feet slowly in ambling fashion. Allow the hands to dangle. Investigate your solar plexus. Is it tense? In case you are not aware of it, it is a big nerve center about two inches above the navel. Relax it. You can do it.

Loosen those neck muscles also. When do they and your solar plexus tighten? When you are angry, worried, or frightened.

To relax, simply refuse to accept any such state of mind. You can do it regardless of your surroundings. I have disciplined my emotions for years, and they have paid me good dividends.

Every time you tell yourself that you can't relax any part of your body you are adding to the tension of the human dynamo up in your skull. No woman ever baked a nice cake the first time she tried, and no man drove a nail straight on his first lick. It takes practice, time after time, and determination to win.

Of course it is much easier to have the masseur or the masseuse help relax your nerves; but what about your pocketbook? If you don't mind that, think about the motor of vour car. If it were hot, you would not turn a fan on it nor throw ice water all over it. You would stop it. That is exactly what I do with my nervous system.

It is true that I give my nerves the best rest at night. Since I have passed seventy I insist on nine hours of relaxed sleeping. You may ask if there is any other kind. There certainly is.

There is the kind in which you are certain before you lie down that you are going to hear the dog next door bark all night; that your husband or wife is going to snore and awaken you; that your son or your daughter is going to come into the living room and you will not sleep another wink all night. How can they care so little about you? You are positive that the jaybird in the tree outside your window will start a racket at daylight and get you up so you cannot get enough rest.

When I lie down on my bed I know that the dog next door *will* bark. He always does, but what of it? It is only my neighbor's dog and will not hurt me nor mine. My husband has snored for years, and I supose he always will. It is noth-

145

ing to worry about, so why even hear it? I don't. I just go to sleep because he is not going to pay any attention if *I* snore. That jaybird outside my window is not going to upset my day either. He is happy, so let something in this old world enjoy itself. The second morning I will not even hear him.

You say it cannot be done? You are right—because so long as you tell yourself you cannot, you will make your words come true. Why not say, "If others can, so can I? If you can do that, you take the first big step toward relaxed sleeping.

Relaxed working under the present tensions is the most difficult care of our nervous systems. A dozen times a day I find my solar plexus tied in a knot which I consciously relax. Try it and see how much better your entire body will feel.